MEDICARE REFORM: THE PRIVATE-SECTOR IMPACT

MEDICARE REFORM: THE PRIVATE-SECTOR IMPACT

AN EBRI-ERF POLICY FORUM

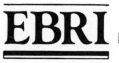 EMPLOYEE BENEFIT RESEARCH INSTITUTE

© 1985 Employee Benefit Research Institute
Education and Research Fund
2121 K Street, NW, Suite 860
Washington, DC 20037-2121
(202) 659-0670

Library of Congress Cataloging-in-Publication Data

Main entry under title:

Medicare reform: the private-sector impact

   "An EBRI-ERF policy forum."
   Forum held June 1985.
   Includes index.
   1. Medicare—Congresses. 2. Insurance, Health—United States—Congresses. I. Salisbury, Dallas L. II. Employee Benefit Research Institute (Washington, D.C.). Education and Research Fund.
HD7102.U4E27   1985   368.4'26'00973   85-25266
ISBN 0-86643-044-X
ISBN 0-86643-045-8 (pbk.)

Printed in the United States of America

Table of Contents

Foreword

As Medicare turns 20, the program is increasingly the target of scrutiny by policymakers and by the elderly citizens who are its intended beneficiaries. Today Medicare is the major program that provides health care protection to the nation's elderly. Nearly 31 million Americans are enrolled in the Medicare program, some 27 million of them age 65 and over.

The primary reason for the rising concern over Medicare has been the well-publicized prediction of a shortfall in Medicare's financing estimated to occur by the end of this century. Yet, Congress in recent years has approached Medicare issues primarily within the context of the federal budget process—and not in any comprehensive attempt to restore long-term solvency to the Medicare system.

With this as background, the Employee Benefit Research Institute undertook to organize a policy forum that would look at Medicare's long-term financing problems from the standpoint of their impact on employers, insurers, health care providers, and consumers, rather than view only their impact on the federal budget.

The need for this kind of analysis remains important despite recent, more optimistic predictions for the short-run solvency of the Medicare program. Even if the short-term situation has improved, the long-term financing deficiency remains acute.

EBRI invited representatives of government, business, consumer and research groups, labor, and the news media to the policy forum, entitled "The Impact of Medicare Reforms on the Private Sector." The forum was held June 6, 1985, in Washington, DC, and consisted of oral presentations by seven distinguished experts, including Rep. Pete Stark of California, chairman of the Health Subcommittee of the House Committee on Ways and Means. A general discussion by participants followed speakers' remarks. A list of the participants appears in Appendix A.

Each speaker invested a major effort in making a substantial contribution to our understanding of Medicare issues. This report contains the edited proceedings of the forum along with papers submitted in advance by several of the speakers.

On behalf of EBRI, I wish to thank the persons who made the policy forum and this book possible: the speakers, the participants, and EBRI staff.

The views expressed in this book are solely those of the speakers and the forum participants. They should not be attributed to the officers, trustees, members, or associates of EBRI, its staff, or its Education and Research Fund.

DALLAS L. SALISBURY
President

October 1985

About the Authors

Fortney H. (Pete) Stark

Rep. Fortney H. (Pete) Stark (D-CA) is chairman of the Subcommittee on Health of the House Committee on Ways and Means. He entered Congress in 1973 and was named to the committee—which deals with taxes, Social Security, health insurance, public assistance, and foreign trade—during his second term. As subcommittee chairman, Stark pledged to "help solve the Medicare financing problem before it becomes a crisis." He holds a bachelor's in engineering from the Massachusetts Institute of Technology and a master's in business administration from the University of California, Berkeley.

Sheila P. Burke

Sheila P. Burke is deputy chief of staff for the Office of the Majority Leader under U.S. Sen. Robert J. Dole (R-KS). She previously served as Dole's deputy staff director at the U.S. Senate Committee on Finance. Burke holds a master's in public administration from Harvard University and a bachelor's in nursing from the University of San Francisco.

Cynthia K. Hosay

Cynthia K. Hosay is national director of health care cost management for the Martin E. Segal Company, and formerly served as director of statewide health programs for the New York State School of Industrial Relations at Cornell University. She earned a master's and a doctorate in community health from New York University.

Stephen H. Long

Stephen H. Long is deputy assistant director for health and income security at the U.S. Congressional Budget Office. He was a tenured associate professor of economics at The Maxwell School at Syracuse University where he had sole responsibility for health economics instruction. Long holds a doctorate in economics from the University of Wisconsin-Madison.

John C. Rother

John C. Rother is associate director for legislation and public policy for the American Association of Retired Persons (AARP). Before joining AARP, Rother served as special counsel for labor and health to former U.S. Sen. Jacob Javits (R-NY) and as staff director and chief counsel for the Special Committee on Aging under its chairman, Sen. John Heinz (R-PA). He is an honors graduate of Oberlin College and the University of Pennsylvania Law School.

John F. Troy

John F. Troy is vice president, corporate communications department, for The Travelers Insurance Companies. He holds a bachelor's in economics from the University of Connecticut and a master's in education from Central Connecticut State University, and earned a law degree from the University of Connecticut.

Karen Williams

Karen Williams is director of research and policy development for the Health Insurance Association of America. Prior to joining HIAA, she was with the Health Care Financing Administration, U.S. Department of Health and Human Services, where she helped design the Medicare prospective payment system for hospitals.

Medicare Reform: What Are the Options?

Remarks of Stephen H. Long

MR. LONG: So much of what I have to say really will not be original, and in fact many of the options CBO [Congressional Budget Office] has laid out recently were prepared before I arrived. So I'm going to make remarks more like a wide-eyed tourist than a seasoned Washingtonian.

I'm trying to keep my remarks at a general level so as not to preempt the other speakers who have specific options they would like to discuss; and in fact, to some extent, I will even drop back and talk more about the basic problem and alternatives, rather than specific options.

A second caveat I would make is that CBO makes no recommendations for policy. So if you hear even the slightest tone of opinion, it was surely me peeking out around my mask of objectivity and not a recommendation of the CBO.

Background on the Issues

It's really hard to design options to solve a problem if you're not quite sure what the problem is, and it's certainly hard to know whether you've succeeded in solving a problem if you don't know what it is. I would like to take just a few minutes to reflect on the nature of the Medicare problem that gives rise to the calls for reform.

Is There a Medicare Crisis?—First let me ask a question. Is there a Medicare crisis? If you polled the newspaper-reading public just a short while ago, I'm sure you'd find the perception that there was a crisis, because the Hospital Insurance (HI) Trust Fund was going broke. If you polled them more recently, you'd probably find that there's not a crisis, because the HI Trust Fund is in good shape. This apparent ambivalence comes about because the projected bankruptcy date keeps moving farther and farther out into the future. A couple of short years ago it was 1987. Then it was 1990. Now, by CBO's latest testimony, it's mid-1990s. The Medicare actuaries have it late 1990s.

This date moves not just because of things we do within the program, but also as a result of a lot of forces that are external to the program. Changes in the general level of prices have a lot to do with

1

it. Trends in utilization, not all of which come about because of policy changes within the program, but as a result of general changes in the health care sector, seem to be changing very rapidly. Employment levels move, and the like.

So one answer to my question is that whether there's a Medicare crisis is very much a function of how prospects for the trust fund look at the moment. These forecasts are very difficult to make. Things change a lot. But I don't think we should dismiss the notion of a basic problem because at the moment there's no trust fund crisis. That doesn't necessarily take away from the spirit of this forum. If HI bankruptcy isn't imminent, there may still be a Medicare problem to be solved.

Now a second answer that's widely known for why there's a Medicare problem, even if HI is not in immediate trouble, is simply because of Supplementary Medical Insurance (SMI), or Part B. It's well known that outlays in Part B continue to rise and, as they rise, they make an automatic call on general revenues to support them. That trust fund doesn't look like it's going broke, due to its design, but SMI has been making a larger and larger share of total outlays in the Medicare program. So that's a second aspect of our problem.

But even if Part B weren't gobbling up general revenues, there is a general federal deficit problem. Medicare outlays contribute mightily to it. Medicare payroll taxes and other revenues represent part of a limited pot of resources that the federal government can tax. In that sense, the Medicare problem will be with us as long as there's a general federal deficit problem and, in fact, much of the current activity in the Congress is a result of this third aspect.

So it's important to go beyond just viewing the trust funds in isolation, but instead to view them as part of the larger federal budget, and in that way we're likely to continue to have a Medicare problem.

Even if there were none of these fiscal pressures, there remain some basic design issues that will arise as the Congress attempts to revise the program to better meet its original goals in the face of change—for example, needs change; technology changes. Those redesigns can include benefit redesign—for example, the issue of catastrophic costs. The cost-sharing issues have changed as private "Medigap" policies have been purchased by a growing share of the elderly. There is always pressure for new benefits, which could range as far as social insurance for long-term care.

In sum, all of these sources of continuing pressure combine to assure us that there will be a need for Medicare reform, and that the problem will be with us for some time to come.

2

Framework for Characterizing the Options—I'd like to discuss a framework for characterizing options for Medicare reform. It's a framework that's been standard in health care financing circles for some time. There are two convenient accounting identities that can be used to characterize and organize options for changing the programs.

The first identity is simply that outlays are the product of the number of eligibles, the average benefits used per eligible, and the average reimbursement rate. That is, bodies times use of services times payments generate total spending on services. Administrative costs can then be tacked on at the end. This describes the factors that determine outlays and the options that are available for lowering their rate of increase: altering the number of bodies, altering the kinds of benefits, or altering what we pay.

On the other hand, there are receipts. The receipt identity can be summarized as beneficiary payments plus taxes equal total receipts.

These identities also highlight the major groups that would be affected by reform. You can see beneficiaries within those identities; likewise, the flow of payments tells you about providers' receipts. Tax payments represent the folks outside the program who are paying in and who, in the long run, may expect to benefit.

Criteria for Assessing the Options—What criteria might be used to assess options? I've identified three commonly mentioned ones that might have some relevance to today's discussion. First, does an option promote the efficient use and provision of health care services? That is, does it promote the least-cost means of providing health services? Do people get what they need and what they're willing to pay for? Second, are benefits or burdens of an option distributed fairly? The groups among whom gains and losses are distributed are beneficiaries, providers, and taxpayers. Third, does a proposed change represent merely a short-run fix or a long-run solution? Now, that's not to say that short-run fixes are undesirable, since sometimes short-run fixes are necessary until one can gather information or data to make long-run, more fundamental changes. But many argue that long-run solutions are needed for long-run problems.

Options

With that background, let me brush quite lightly across a range of options that seem to be possible for Medicare change. Some of them are short-run, but many are long-run. There were a number of particular CBO options distributed in the packets to participants. [See

3

Appendix D.] I won't go over the details of those particular options here. They include cost or savings estimates, some discussion of how they might work, and a discussion of their advantages and disadvantages. They come from a standard CBO product that is distributed annually with alternative ways to reduce the federal budget.

Eligibility—If we consider the accounting identity for outlays, the list of options can begin with eligibility. Now, eligibility is a tough one, because you are looking at a program that comes out of a long social insurance history, and many would argue that the essentially universal eligibility for the elderly under the Medicare program is something that has a long tradition. They would argue that this tradition should be upheld. Fine-tuning around that eligibility is really a matter of retirement policy. It certainly goes beyond Medicare alone. The big options in eligibility have to do with changing the retirement age or the eligibility age as ways of delaying payout. In contrast, smaller changes include those in provisions that affect working elderly. Eligibility policy has not, however, been the main focus of activity. That is because they involve far more fundamental changes in the assumptions of the program.

Benefits—Turning to benefits, some of the key options have to do with redesigning toward providing more catastrophic benefits. But with concern about the budget, these options are usually tied to some offsetting form of savings. A common version of this option would expand benefits for catastrophic illness, but impose more cost sharing at the front end of care across a wider set of people as an offset to the cost.

A longer-term issue in benefits is how the society deals with long-term care concerns—that is, whether we continue to leave long-term care out in the Medicaid and private arena or bring it under a possible Medicare "Part C." This would be a major redesign of benefits, a long-term thing. It's obviously not on the current agenda.

Reimbursement—Since changing the benefit structure is not a major source of savings, most of the near-term options and most of the long-term concern come on the reimbursement side.

Obviously, major change has recently been made in the way we pay hospitals. For the near term, there are several options for adjusting the prospective payment system [PPS] and other forms of payment to hospitals that are not covered within the diagnosis-related group [DRG] rates. Issues include questions of timing the move to a national rate; wage indexing; paying for graduate medical education, both the direct and the indirect components; hospitals serving a disproportionate share of low-income people; and paying

4

for hospital capital. All of these near-term issues and options involve a good deal of concern about equity of treatment across the different types of hospitals and a lot of uncertainty because the data systems are so far behind. We have so little information on what has happened since PPS started that it's difficult to know whether the system is moving in the expected direction of greater efficiency or not. The data gap hampers attempts to say what the implications of various changes will be.

Although the near-term issues for the prospective payment system all can involve substantial shifts in dollars, they pale in comparison to the longer-term issues of how the rate of aggregate growth in payment should be determined. Small changes in the proportion of market-basket increases that are allowed to feed into higher DRG rates have big effects on the trust fund well into the future. Effectively, the system has changed from paying on costs to giving central control over the total payment to hospitals. The biggest problem here is gauging how fast the system can be pushed toward efficiency.

On Part B, Supplementary Medical Insurance, there are short-term freezes in physician payment, whereas in the longer run there are issues of reform. The options all involve issues of how to design systems that will control the volume and not just the price that physicians are paid for each unit of service. Most approaches look to ways of bundling procedures so that larger groups of services can be paid for in single payments and in that way attempt to control a physician's discretion over the volume of services recommended. The two kinds of options that seem to get the most consideration here are fee schedules and physician DRGs. Under fee schedules there is a variety of options on how to set up relative values schedules, set the prices, and vary them over time. Under physician DRG payments the research literature seems to suggest that there may be some possibilities in surgery. Physician DRGs for medical care, instead, are a more difficult option to design. I think the research literature is far more cautious about the ability to implement the latter form.

Financing—Turning away from the outlay side, the options on the financing side can be classified by where additional revenues will come from. Despite all attempts to control outlays, there's little question that they will go up; so from where will the financing come? Globally, financing is derived from two groups—beneficiaries and taxpayers. So, at a global level the options involve answering the questions of intergenerational equity, then, within those two groups, deciding who should pay and how much.

On the beneficiary side, many are looking at the rising economic

5

status of the elderly and suggesting that beneficiaries might be asked to contribute more. Others are arguing that the elderly should be protected. The options for the longer run, if beneficiaries were to be asked to pay more, tend to revolve around issues of income-related contributions. If increased burdens are to be borne by beneficiaries, there is a concern for the low-income ones among them. This concern arises in two ways: first, their ability to pay increased amounts, but second, concerns about them staying within the system, continuing to pay premiums for Part B rather than dropping out. The options for income-related financing in premiums tend to piggyback on the income-tax system for administrative convenience. Other options for charging beneficiaries involve taxing Medigap policies. The rationale is that ownership of Medigap insurance increases utilization because cost sharing is covered by insurance, and the increased use imposes costs on the program. The rationale for taxing premiums is for the program to recapture some of that extra spending.

If, instead, financing is to come from taxpayers, there is a variety of options. Payroll taxes can be increased, further general revenues can be tapped, or special taxes on particular commodities might be raised. The ones that get a lot of consideration include alcohol and tobacco taxes.

Administration—Stepping back from these various options, another issue that many are talking about is an administrative issue—the separation of Parts A and B. The current arrangement causes some difficulty in data availability for assessing the program. Particularly as options involve cutting back on particular portions in either A or B, there are concerns about spillovers or behavioral shifts that are difficult to track because of the separate recordkeeping and the like. An example is current concern about fair reimbursement across substitute sites—that is, surgical reimbursement across inpatient, outpatient, and ambulatory surgery centers. Some have argued that the separation of the two trust funds is an artificial one and that merging them would provide administrative convenience, data convenience, and, ultimately, evaluation convenience.

I'll leave it to the other speakers to move on to more specific details on these options.

Where Will the Emphasis Be in Congress and the Administration?

Remarks of Sheila P. Burke

MS. BURKE: I'd like to build a little bit on what Steve Long has laid out for you, which I think is probably a good overview of the options that are being considered by the Congress.

I think, if nothing else, you can certainly say that there don't appear to be any easy solutions or any particularly new solutions. It's really a question of a balancing among all the options that are being laid before us.

I think it is also safe to say that, in the short term—as we've seen really since 1980, having gone through OBRA and TEFRA and DEFRA [the Omnibus Budget Reconciliation Act of 1981, the Tax Equity and Fiscal Responsibility Act of 1982, and the Deficit Reduction Act of 1984, respectively] and a few of the other bills in recent years—to a certain extent we're going to be budget-driven in terms of our priorities.

In the past, the [finance] committee, at least on the Senate side, really looked to the opportunity of budget reconciliation to try and do both reductions in terms of spending reductions or cost-saving kinds of activities.

So I would simply say that whatever you're likely to see done in terms of the short term is likely to be done in the context of the budget rather than big reform bills moving through separately.

Congressional Priorities

Now, in looking at the committee's priorities—and again, having left the committee, I can only say it from the perception of somebody who's sort of looking from the outside—I would probably divide it into three areas. The three are: institutional providers, individual providers, and beneficiary changes. I would further split them into two areas.

One would be reimbursement reform and the second, benefit reform. With respect to reimbursement reform, I think it should come as no surprise to anybody who's been tracking this for the last couple of years that there continues to be an awful lot of interest and a lot

7

of activity in looking at further changes to the system that has been developed over the last two to three years.

There's an awful lot of pressure—particularly with respect to institutional providers, but I think it's also true with respect to physician providers, as Steve Long has pointed out—to try and bundle as many things as possible and to try and continue to tinker to a certain extent with the kinds of programs that have recently been put into place.

With respect to institutional providers and reimbursement reform, there's no doubt that a lot of time is going to be spent looking at what's going on with respect to DRGs: one, with respect to the things that were not incorporated the first time around; for example, institutions and units that were not covered, pediatric institutions, rehabilitation institutions, things of that nature; but also looking at the kinds of tinkering that we need to do to make the system work a little better.

With respect to the institutional providers that weren't included, we are continuing to struggle, both the administration and the Congress, with trying to fit them into that DRG mold.

There is no doubt there are problems with doing that. Both pediatric institutions and rehabilitation institutions don't seem to fit as easily into a DRG kind of a system.

There's a lot of work being done. How quickly that will be resolved is not clear. I don't think it's going to be in the short term.

Adjusting for Severity

With respect to tinkering with the other pieces of the system, clearly at the top of the list is severity.

We've talked about that repeatedly since the beginning of the DRG program. It is something that everyone would like to do, and no one seems yet to know how best to do it.

There's work, obviously, taking place across the country. I'm sure a lot of you are aware of that work, particularly that of Johns Hopkins University, trying to look at a number of options including disease staging systems, something that lets us look a little more closely at the actual case that's being cared for, and try to adjust to the extent that they fall outside of the average. The outlier policy [i.e., additional payment for atypical cases] that was originally put into place was in part a short-term solution to that problem.

Again, I don't think that's going to be a short-term kind of issue. I think that we've not yet found an easy way to adjust for severity without returning to cost-based reimbursement, which no one is in a big hurry to do, at least as far as the Congress is concerned. But the closer you get to trying to make it more sensitive, the closer you risk going back to cost.

Indigent Care

The other big issue, obviously, that hangs out there is indigent care. Some of that, to a certain extent, is wrapped up in the severity issue. No doubt about it. There will be those who argue—and have, I think, argued quite reasonably over the last few years—that people who come from lower socio-economic groups tend to be sicker and tend to bring bigger problems to the institution where they're cared for. They tend not to have the kind of social system that supports them in going home as quickly. It has been argued that institutions bear additional costs because of this type of population. We continue to struggle with trying to quantify what that difference is and trying to figure out a way to represent that difference in our payment model.

There is also, however, a separate discussion taking place with respect to that issue. Should Medicare share in the cost of caring for individuals who are not Medicare beneficiaries?

There are clearly two issues here. One is the question of the low-income elderly who are Medicare beneficiaries and whether, in fact, they are sicker and whether institutions that care for those individuals incur higher costs because of (1) the severity of the illness and (2) their socio-economic status.

The second issue is really a question of what to do with those individuals who are non-Medicare and indigent and those who are disenfranchised from the work force, have no third-party payment, and are not eligible for Medicaid.

To what extent should Medicare get into that business? This, I think, will be one of the most difficult things for us to deal with.

Institutions, particularly large public institutions, are successfully, I think, raising these issues before the Congress to try and get some kind of a resolution of this question.

Institutional Reform

This year, I suspect, there are no great surprises in terms of the budget legislation with respect to institutions. Again, I don't think you're going to see any major reforms or major adjustments in the system.

A one-year freeze of the DRG payment rates has been proposed. I suspect the issue that will accompany the one-year freeze is whether or not the transition ought to be frozen and how quickly, in fact, we ought to move toward a national rate. There are those who would argue that if you, in fact, freeze the rates, you ought to freeze the entire system in place for that period of time. There are others who clearly benefit from the movement to a national rate who are anxious not to have that process slowed down. So I suspect that you will see that issue fought out in the committees of jurisdiction.

There are other kinds of changes on the institutional side that will be fought out, again, in the short term and then over the long term in terms of policy; one is medical education and the role Medicare should play with respect to the financing of graduate medical education and the education of nonphysician providers—for example, the contribution to nursing education that takes place in an institutional setting.

Again, you're seeing two battles taking place. One is the bigger battle which is, should Medicare have any role whatsoever? Then the question: if, in fact, it has a role, how significant should that role be, and should Medicare play a role in terms of distribution of manpower?

There are some of us who would argue that, in fact, Medicare's business is not manpower distribution policy. We ought not to be in the business of saying you ought to have "X" number of internists versus "X" number of surgeons. But there are also those who would argue that, in fact, by supporting certain kinds of specialties, Medicare runs the risk of higher and higher outlays. Many believe that to the extent you support subspecialties, you risk tremendous expenditures in the out years.

Medical Education

The Finance Committee recently held a hearing on financing of direct medical education. I suspect we'll also be visiting the subject of indirect expenditures.

The Senate-passed budget resolution contains a savings estimate that assumes a reduction in the indirect adjustment. It's a straight budget cut. There's no particular policy reform that's reflected in terms of that particular proposal which was also in the administration's package. However, the Congress, when they agreed to the DRGs, took the position that the indirect medical education adjustment was a proxy for severity to a certain extent. As a result, until we could solve severity, we agreed to double the teaching adjustment in an attempt to deal with some of those large tertiary institutions and try and address some of their concerns.

The administration's position is that there is no basis upon which we should double that teaching adjustment. Therefore, in the absence of any data, we should simply reduce it to where it was. I suspect the Congress may take some issue with that assumption, because they doubled it for a specific reason, and that reason has not been addressed.

Over the long term, again, I think we'll question what role Medicare should play with respect to medical education expenses, both direct and indirect. Again, there is the question of whether Medicare patient dollars ought to be used to support individuals who tend to come out with fairly high incomes, who have other alternatives for financing their education, either through loans or scholarships, and the institutions themselves, which can look to faculty practice plans and perhaps other options in terms of revenues to try and support those teaching programs. I think there's likely to be a struggle.

Reimbursement

Over the long term, with respect to reimbursement reform, I think there's a lot of pressure to try and group as many of the services into that payment as possible. With respect to smaller institutions—for example, skilled nursing facilities [SNFs] and home health agencies—there are those who would argue that payment ought to reflect the total continuum of care from the point of admission to discharge to post-hospital care. Needless to say, neither the nursing home industry nor the home health agencies are anxious to have the hospitals given all of those dollars.

There are those, however, who argue that until you get that full range of services incorporated into that payment, there's discrimination among the benefits and you can't really control the total case costs for that particular client.

There is a certain amount of this coordination already going. Institutions, particularly large hospitals, are getting into the business of providing home health care and even nursing home services more so than they used to. They're certainly getting into the long-term care business, which causes the nursing home industry a lot of heartburn. The "swing bed" concept that was incorporated in 1980 is a piece of that. The so-called swing bed concept was an attempt to solve a problem in rural areas where there tend to be very few skilled nursing

11

facilities and 100-percent occupancies in those that are available. As a result of DRGs, when people are being discharged on a quicker basis and you have no place to put them, you run a tremendous amount of risk.

As a result there's a lot of support for making sure nursing home beds are available in the community. But in defense of the nursing home industry, Medicare really hasn't revisited its reimbursement policy with respect to skilled nursing facilities. We're not really paying for heavy-care patients in skilled nursing facilities.

There's no doubt about it. There's no adjustment or recognition for the fact that those patients are sicker, and increasingly so as the acuity goes up as a result of earlier discharges. So we really owe it to the industry and to ourselves to spend some time looking at what's happening on the long-term care side, looking at ways to make that reimbursement system make more sense so that those individuals and institutions are in the business of trying to care for heavier-care patients.

I think there is an interest on the industry side in trying to get some kind of a prospective payment for long-term care, for skilled care, if possible. That's a difficult thing to do. We know even less, in many ways, about those costs and how they fit into either diagnosis relationships with the DRGs or some other mechanism and what the indicators ought to be in terms of resource utilization.

When you get a patient whose average length of stay is 30, 60, or 90 days in the long-term care facility, it's tough to try and decide what payment model makes more sense. But I think there's a lot of pressure to try and address each of those pieces.

Home Health Care

On the home care or home health agency side, there are a whole range of issues that need addressing. One, again, is the question of what Medicare's role ought to be with respect to the provision of home health services. To what extent should we limit our exposure to health- or medical-related services and not custodial care or non-health-related services? Keeping people at home isn't cheap. It's cheaper than keeping them in a large, acute care hospital, perhaps in an ICU [intensive care unit] bed, but it's not inexpensive to maintain people at home.

There are questions as to whether or not we ought to re-examine that benefit, given again the pressures under DRGs to get people home, to keep them out of institutions—whether we ought to rethink what Medicare's role ought to be.

The administration has seemed to approach this on a confrontational basis in terms of trying to force as many issues as they can with respect to home health agency services—an increased number of denials with respect to those benefits or a questioning of the homebound requirement, the intermittent care requirement. We have fought over that for the last couple of years.

I would suspect, of any of these areas, home care is likely to see the largest range of administrative changes, continuing to try and push the answers to those questions in terms of what Medicare's responsibility ought to be.

My sense is that the Congress is at some point going to get involved in a major way in trying to rethink the home health benefit. Frankly, I don't think we have. We've avoided for a long time, at least in the Finance Committee, getting into the long-term care debate and the home health care debate, in a way, frankly, because I don't think we knew what to do.

It's much harder to define or resolve that question than it is to resolve big institutional questions. But I suspect there's going to be growing pressure for us to look at that piece of the benefit, again as a result of all these other changes and the changes in the incentives in the system.

Individual Provider Reimbursement

With respect to individual providers, and physicians in particular, I think Steve Long did an excellent job of laying out for you the range of options that people are looking at, from physician DRGs to fee schedules.

Again, I think there are two things going on. One is an attempt to try and control our exposure, to try and begin to address the rapid escalation in Part B expenditures, to try and package services into larger and larger groups, including those provided by physicians, and to try and control the total cost—and, on the other side, to try and put some equity into the system. I think if anyone has made a good case it's been the internists who, over the last couple of years, have argued that they are, in fact, discriminated against by the present payment model which they argue, in fact, benefits those technological services that we've seen grow over the last few years, and as a result tend to benefit the surgeons, people who do "things" or specific procedures.

13

That's not surprising; that's the history of the reimbursement system under Part B. But there's a lot of interest in trying to address that problem so that you remove some of the disincentives to the provision of ambulatory care services that are less costly in many cases than institutional services.

I think, again, there are two things that are going to take place. In the short term, I don't think you're going to see major reimbursement reform, in part because I think we again don't yet know what direction we ought to take.

I think the broad range of options that CBO has looked at, the administration is looking at—the report that is due to us in July [1985]—are all going to attempt to lay out what the pros and cons are of all of those options.

Again, as Steve Long pointed out, there seems to be a much higher chance of doing things on the inpatient surgical side than there is on the ambulatory side, which is very difficult to deal with. I think it's safe to say, however, that there does not seem to be overwhelming support for DRGs for physicians.

There is overwhelming support for some kind of reform, but I don't think anyone's really coalesced around one particular option. I think people are interested in looking at the implications of certain kinds of changes. One of the reasons we're interested in doing that is, frankly, Medicare has been very successful at keeping the elderly in mainstream medicine. The large majority of physicians are still willing to care for Medicare patients. We are having a tremendous response for the participating physician program. We can debate the reasons why, but there is certainly a dramatic increase in the number of assigned claims. I think we're going to be looking at that, trying to understand what the implications are of that kind of a system.

The assignment issue continues to be one that troubles people and will certainly be the subject of a lot of debate around any reimbursement reform proposal. The question is whether we ought to require that physicians, like institutions, accept assignment and, therefore, protect the beneficiary from out-of-pocket costs beyond what they anticipate.

I think physicians, particularly some of the specialty groups, are also very actively involved in trying to find solutions to these problems; but there are those who, no doubt, will bring every force to bear that they can to try and block any kind of reimbursement change on the physician side.

In some ways, I think it will be more difficult than it was on the hospital side, but I think that there's an awful lot of pressure in the right kind of environment to accomplish physician reimbursement reform. If anything has been dramatic in the last few years, it's been watching the changing attitude of the Congress and their willingness to take on physicians, and I think that that is as true today and perhaps will become increasingly true over the next couple of years.

There's just enormous frustration with the sort of mentality that argues for status quo, recognizing the kinds of problems we're having with physician reimbursement.

So I think there will be progress in that area. In the short term, I think it's likely to be a continuation of some kind of freeze. I think Mr. Waxman[1] is looking at options that try to hold down certain kinds of fees. The Senate has suggested that we carve out those physicians who have been willing to participate, to try and provide them with some recognition of their willingness to do so.

I'm sure the elderly groups will be anxious to try and look at what the risks are for the beneficiary, in looking at the extension of that freeze; but I think that there's some support, if you're going to freeze the rest of the system, to try and again maintain some kind of control with respect to physician reimbursement.

Beneficiary Reform

With respect to beneficiaries, the last major group of issues, in the short term, again, I don't think you're likely to see any major changes. You'll see continued tinkering with the deductible and cost-sharing relationships.

Again, it was suggested this year—it's not clear what the outcome will be—to try and place some cost-sharing requirements on the home health benefit, again, a relooking at the premium and whether the Medicare beneficiary ought to pay a higher percentage of the premium.

The same old fight—it began at 50 percent of the program's cost. It declined to about 23 percent. We fixed it at 25 percent. Now there is a suggestion that it go back up to a higher percentage.

In that issue, however, and in all of the beneficiary issues, there is the continuing concern with respect to the low-income elderly and how you protect them against increased cost sharing that puts them at risk in terms of lack of access to services or inability to finance services.

---

[1]Editor's note: U.S. Rep. Henry A. Waxman (D-CA) is chairman of the Health and Environment Subcommittee of the House Committee on Energy and Commerce, and a member of the House Select Committee on Aging.

One answer is that some of them are, in fact, picked up under Medicaid and, therefore, cost sharing is taken care of, but that's not true for all of them. There's a group of them that fall out of that system, folks that are right on the line; and there's a lot of concern about trying to protect those individuals.

Over the long term, again I think, as Steve Long correctly pointed out, there will be a tremendous pressure to look at the beneficiary's long-term role with respect to Medicare. There's been some tinkering to try and encourage people to stay in the private insurance market— the working-aged provisions that were enacted a couple of years ago. We first began, if you remember, with the ESRD [end-stage renal disease] program, to try and get some of the ESRD benefit back on the private side, then the working-aged provision for people that stayed in the work force, and then a further expansion being suggested this year.

So there's one question, which is to try and keep them on the private side as long as you can, and then the other question is, for those who do go into Medicare, whether, given the resources that are available to Medicare over the long term, you ought to rethink what happens with respect to the high-income beneficiary.

Now the example that's always used, which is the extreme example, is, why should we pay for a Rockefeller under the Medicare program when they're fully capable of paying for those services with some other means? But the Rockefellers are the very small percentage of the population. So I don't think that's the honest argument to use. But there will be questions about whether or not there are certain elderly who are able to finance more services out of their pocket, therefore allowing us a target for the remaining funds.

The difficulty in that argument will be the introduction of means testing, the introduction of a welfare philosophy with respect to a program that has been seen historically as not a social welfare benefit but as a retirement benefit, one that doesn't really raise the question of income and whether people ought to be eligible on the basis of income. That will be a very difficult issue, but I think again, because of the dwindling resources of the trust fund and concern about low-income elderly, there will be attention given to that particular issue.

Increasing Revenues

The last major group of issues are really the revenue issues. Again, Steve Long touched on a broad range of these.

This year, I suspect, the two that hold out some possibility in terms of debates in the Congress are, one, the expansion of coverage to include state and local workers—that's the one group that still remains outside of the system. Mandatory coverage would provide a good chunk of money to the trust fund. There are about 70 percent of state and local workers who are already covered under the Medicare system, so it's just the expansion to cover on a mandatory basis those remaining populations.

The other is the dedication of a tax. Again, as has been suggested, the cigarette and alcohol taxes have been most frequently mentioned. But I suspect that there will be those who are less willing to do that, if you're going to do it and not put it into general revenues for deficit reduction rather than into a trust fund. I think that there is little or no support for an increase in the payroll tax. I think there are mixed reactions to the introduction of general-revenue financing into Part A.

Of course, Part B is already 75-percent financed by general revenues, but with the introduction of general revenues into Part A—there are those who would argue that you lose some control or some sense of control, because of the nature of a trust fund where you have a limited number of dollars. There are those who would argue that you really don't have a lot of general revenues to pump into anything anyway. There are no extra dollars floating around.

I don't think you're likely, otherwise, to see any big changes with respect to revenues this year. Again, I think, as the impending insolvency of the fund has been pushed farther and farther back, the Congress is not about to take on a fight it doesn't have to take on, particularly this close to an election. Those of you who would argue that we've just gotten through one don't realize that we started running for 1986 about four months ago. So we're already looking at people talking about a mentality of an election year.

You're likely to see some tinkering. I don't think you're likely to see any major pushes for reimbursement reform in the short term.

Perhaps you will see us try and resolve some of the remaining PPS issues, with some debate going on over the longer term with respect to things that we can do maybe next year or post-election 1986 and maybe 1987 when we're getting ready for 1988.

Discussion

Psychiatric Care

MR. KITTREDGE: I may have missed it, but I don't recall hearing any mention of psychiatric care in the list of institutions that are not now controlled and where there's pretty strong evidence that the facilities for psychiatric care are expanding in leaps and bounds.

MS. BURKE: You're right, Jack. I didn't mention it. It is again one of the institutions or groups of services left out. The same problem is true with respect to psych benefits that is true of rehab and pediatrics: that is, trying to find whether there's any basis for a reimbursement system that tries to group services and set an average price. In psych, particularly, and also rehab, there is a problem in terms of the length of treatment, that people tend to stay for long periods of time.

With pediatrics we just have so little exposure. I mean, it's not as much of an issue. I think it's just the nature of a psych benefit that makes it so hard to define and try and put people into groups in terms of resource utilization. The American Psychiatric Association, the psychiatric hospitals, and others are working with the administration to try and sort that out; but I don't think that's moving along terribly quickly either.

It raises an interesting question, one that we've begun and sort of goes into the benefit reform side, that is, re-examining what Medicare ought to be financing. The question we are asking—because Senator [Robert J.] Dole asked me to start pursuing it—is whether or not we ought to re-examine the kind of internal controls on the Medicare psych benefit.

Now we have a bizarre limit on the outpatient side of about $250. We are asking whether we ought to try and trade some of the inpatient for the outpatient to try and expand the use of ambulatory services, particularly given the growth of the kind of services that are available on an ambulatory basis. Now, I don't know that we can find an easy way to do that trade-off, but I think there's interest in trying to expand the use of ambulatory care.

There's always been this real fear of the psych benefit—you know, that once you sort of stick a toe in, you're going to get dragged in completely. We had scream therapists testify one year, and a whole range of interesting people testify on the psych benefit. It's one of Jay

Constantine's[1] favorite subjects right after HMOs [health maintenance organizations].

I mean, there's a lot of concern; but I think there's also an acceptance that psych services aren't going to go away. Maybe we ought
to try and do something about it.

MR. KITTREDGE: Matter of fact, if anything, it's going to become a
bigger problem.

MS. BURKE: Yes. I think we're also looking to the private sector
where you seem to have moved a little more quickly than we have
in an acceptance of psychiatric services and certain kinds of therapies,
and on doing so devised internal limits, maybe that make a little
more sense.

MR. KITTREDGE: Doesn't mean it's any easier to control.

MS. BURKE: No. No, absolutely. I think that's why we're so concerned.

Program Financing

MR. SEIDMAN: I think it was you, Sheila, who mentioned a figure
on the percentage of the total expenditures of the program that are
covered by general revenue and the trend in that. But I think a relevant figure which ought to be kept in mind is the percentage of
expenditure which comes from out-of-pocket costs of the beneficiaries.

MS. BURKE: —that Medicare does not pay for.

MR. SEIDMAN: And that figure, amazingly, is as high now as before
Medicare was enacted.

MS. BURKE: That's correct.

MR. SEIDMAN: I think that should also be kept in mind.

MS. BURKE: —the percentage of income that the elderly spend.

MR. SEIDMAN: I mean, then you get into the question as to means
testing and so on, and I have my position on that. But I think just in
terms of a relevant figure, we should keep that in mind.

---

[1]Editor's note: Jay Constantine is a former principal staff member for health issues
of the Senate Committee on Finance; he is now a private consultant.

MS. BURKE: You're absolutely right. The percentage of income the elderly spend on health services is similar to what it was in 1965. There are a broad range of things that are not covered at all.

MR. HARRINGTON: Is that primarily due to frequency of expense claims or level of expense, relative to income?

MR. BURKE: That's, I believe, in real-dollar terms, the percentage.

MR. HARRINGTON: We don't know if it constitutes higher utilization? I'm just saying, of the two components, which is having the more significant influence? Does it constitute more care as a percentage of their income, or is it just the dollar relationship?

MS. BURKE: Both, I would argue; I think, probably, particularly given the intensity of services. Probably both.

Physicians' Charges

MR. DETLEFS: The doubling of the number of physicians in this country during the past 20 years doesn't seem to have had the usual supply/demand effect on their charges. To maintain their incomes, maybe some have just decided to cut more often or something, I don't know. But don't we have to move toward some DRG system?

You say that's difficult. Perhaps it requires some other type of prospective payment system, both in the private sector and in Medicare, to control these charges better, because that's a major part of the cost problem. Physicians generally still have very high incomes.

MS. BURKE: I think there are two issues. One is the unit of payment. I mean, what unit of payment makes sense. The other question is the volume control.

Those who argue in support of organizations like HMOs, where you have capitated fees, argue that there's pressure on both volume and on the unit cost for services, and that that kind of a capitated model that incorporates the full range of services is the only way to really get things under control, because the provider is at risk. The more they do, the more it costs them, in effect; rather than the reverse of the fee-for-service model, the more you do, the more you get.

So I think that there is pressure to try and address both of those issues. You're right. The number of things that are provided has expanded rapidly, and I think there's pressure to try and look at both of those in trying to do reimbursement reform.

It is not clear to people that DRGs are the only option, however, in part because of the difficulty, particularly on the ambulatory side, of fitting all those services into particular units of payment—whether that makes sense.

Questions are raised about who gets those dollars—I mean, the kind of technical issues you have to address. If it's a medical case, do you give it to the admitting physician or the primary-care physician? Who do the dollars go to? Do you give it to the hospital, if it's an inpatient service? What do you do on an outpatient basis, particularly with chronic care, people that are cared for over long periods of time?

It's just more difficult to do with physicians than it is with institutions where you have a finite service. You're admitted; you're cared for; you're discharged. It's tougher to do with physicians, but you're absolutely right. There are those who argue that you have to get some payment that encapsulates both of those things so you can control cost and volume of services.

Means Testing

MS. LEWIN: We talk frequently these days about the growing prosperity of the elderly, specifically about their growing assets and income. Given this new reality, there is considerable thought being given to means testing Medicare. Do you think it's doable, feasible?

MS. BURKE: I don't know. I mean, I think the technical question is how best to do it—whether you do it through the tax side, whether you do it through a premium. Trying to do it at the point of purchase has been seen by everybody as being terribly difficult, to try and require a provider to actually do income testing.

So I think there are the technical issues that will have to be resolved. The others are the political issues. I don't know whether we can reach resolution on that. There are those who will fight vigorously against any introduction of an income or means test into a system that was not designed as a welfare system. The real fear is that it will turn into a Medicaid kind of system and, therefore, lose a lot of its public and provider support.

Again, on the other side, I think there are those who would argue that if you're going to have a dwindling number of resources, you ought to target them on the people that need them the most, and that the way to do that is to try and introduce some kind of means testing.

Now the question will be whether it's means testing through cost sharing or means testing through eligibility. My sense is, of those two, it's more likely to be in terms of cost sharing and not eligibility, which would tie it even more tightly to the Medicaid model, which we want to avoid.

I think the question is whether the elderly can pay more out of pocket. In the last couple of years there have been those on the Finance Committee who have publicly stated a position in support of trying to do that. I think they're not going to take that issue on before they have to. When they have to, if the Social Security trust fund or Medicare is in trouble, they're likely to do the same thing they did with Social Security cash—try and reach some kind of compromise. With respect to Social Security, the Congress introduced a method of recapture in terms of taxing certain individuals as part of the Social Security Amendments of 1983.

The Congress has taken a step towards means testing. Now, whether they're willing to carry it over to Medicare—I don't know the answer to that question.

Cost Sharing

MR. HARRINGTON: Sheila, if as a matter of fact, say, 60 percent of expenses are associated with the terminal stages of life, and if this percent is, as I have indicated, the majority of expense, then cost sharing there isn't going to make a difference in most cases.

MS. BURKE: No. One would argue it would not. I mean, that's been a debate about catastrophic illness. If you provide catastrophic care, a catastrophic benefit, what choices do people really have in terms of cost sharing? The question is whether you ought to do it at that point or whether you should do it before in terms of trying to discourage utilization of—

MR. HARRINGTON: Then doesn't it become more of a question of setting?

MS. BURKE: It does become a question of setting. I mean, that's why there's been pressure to move people out of institutions to ambulatory settings as much as possible. Absolutely. So that you end up with tertiary institutions really caring for just the sickest individuals and try and do things on a less costly basis with the others. Absolutely.

Medicare and the Federal Budget

MR. MERRILL: Both of you said, and we hear this all the time, that we can't make any real changes in Medicare now because we're dealing with the budget issue, that the focus is on reducing the deficit, not so much on Medicare. That sort of implies that when the budget

23

issues go away, we'll make some changes in Medicare. The alternative—and this is the question—is: is it possible that when the budget issues go away, Medicare will go away, too, as a policy issue? So the only real hope is while the budget issues are there that some changes might be made?

Ms. BURKE: I guess I wouldn't argue that no reform will take place because of the budget. I mean, if you look at what we've done since 1980, there have been dramatic changes in the program since 1980, all in the context of budget. I guess what I was trying to argue was that we are, in fact, budget-driven. And the activity will take place to a large extent around that process, around the reconciliation process.

You will see, I think, continued changes. I don't think you'll see massive reform until we're forced to do so because of Medicare solvency. That may well still be in the context of a budget. You're absolutely right. I think that those things will continue to go along hand in hand.

I don't think the budget changes are in the absence of policy. I think there's a lot of policy change taking place, but it's taking place in the context of what is being defined as budget kinds of fights rather than big reform fights. Change happens; but I think it's happening in a bigger fight over the budget generally.

MR. LONG: I guess my argument was that I think the budget thing is certainly a long-term thing. It's not going to go away right away, I think. So that that really does drive not only these short-term needs but then large things like physician reimbursement and what-not will eventually come to the fore after some smaller things have been handled. My point was more that, as the concern about the trust fund disappears, there's still plenty of pressure from the budget situation.

Quality of Care

MR. JACKSON: I'm concerned about the quality of medical care for people. One observation that I've made over the years, and I think many people would agree with me, is that when the government steps in to control costs, rent control being one good illustration, short term you'll end up controlling things. Long term, you end up with secondary effects. Landlords don't keep up apartments. New buildings aren't built, and so on. In this area, I've heard a lot of discussion about the practice of medicine and how people ought to be bunching things this way or that way.

I'm not a doctor, but I don't think very many of the people on the U.S. Senate Finance Committee are doctors either. So I wonder whether as a nation, in the long run, having the financial controls there enabling the government to get into more and more details that start dictating methods of treatment and so on is really the best way to improve medical care.

Short run, I can see many of these solutions working. Long run, if you get deeply enough into the practice of medicine, you can make it such an unattractive field that all of our bright young people won't become doctors. I just wonder to what extent, in developing these short-run solutions, anybody is worried about the long-run effect.

You can land on the doctors today, because some of them are overcharging. When you land on them with a bill that controls everything that they do, bright young people looking for careers look at that and say, I don't want to do that. I want to do something else. Then we end up with a collection of people who are doctors who might well have been plumbers at one point, but they're the only people left who want to get into medical school.

Ms. Burke: I don't think we run any short-term risk of people dropping out of medicine for fear of a drop in income.

You're absolutely correct. There are no physicians on the Senate Finance Committee. There are, however, a number of former patients on the Senate Finance Committee who have had a fair amount of experience with the system, my boss being a good example, being someone who was hospitalized for three years. I think Bob Dole is somewhat sensitive to quality in terms of service delivery. And we hear a lot from constituents. We also hear from the AMA [American Medical Association] every time they testify that we can't do anything because it will radically alter the quality of care.

That argument is an important one, but I'm not sure it's one that ought to prevent us from doing anything to make more sense out of the system, because we also hear the arguments from consumers about inappropriate services because of the nature of the reimbursement system that encourage people to do more to get more—unnecessary services, unnecessary surgery. You know, I think that there are arguments on both sides about trying to get a handle on the kinds of services that we're providing.

The PSRO [Professional Standards Review Organization] or PRO [Peer Review Organization] program is not the solution to all of those kinds of issues, and it's an attempt to try and get at some of those questions. But the difficulty in quality is in defining what it is that you mean by quality and trying to put into place some system that monitors quality. Now, I think the elderly groups and their attempts to try and participate actively in those programs on a local and state-wide basis are a critical piece of that.

I think the best person to comment is the person who's received the service if they're given the ability to do so through some kind of a mechanism where their comments are understood and taken into account.

I don't think that the Congress is ignorant of the fact that there are quality questions. There are a lot of people who are concerned that DRGs by the nature of the payment model will, in fact, encourage institutions to do as little as possible. They're the same people who were, I would argue, concerned about HMOs because of the PHP [prepaid health plan] scandal in the 1970s in California, concerned about HMOs only being in the business of providing as little as they could and keeping all the dollars.

So what you do is, as you go along, you try and address those concerns with each kind of change. Severity, the whole question of an index for severity, is an attempt to address that issue, to try and make sure that there are adequate resources to, in fact, provide services that are necessary.

I would argue that institutions and the public generally have no appreciation of the value of nursing services in hospitals. And, therefore, the DRGs really don't adequately address nursing resource allocation, which is the single most or the largest component of services provided to an individual in a hospital. So we really need to look and talk with those from nursing service to try and understand that more clearly.

Now I think we're all going through an ongoing process of understanding, and of trying to address quality questions as they come to the forefront. So I think it is understating the position of the Congress to suggest that they don't, in fact, understand or appreciate quality. I think that's a very important question to all of them, and I think we're all trying to struggle with it, as is the community at large.

I mean, medicine is trying to understand it. Nursing is trying to understand it. Hospital administrators are trying to understand it. I think we're all in the business of trying to do the best we can with what we have available to us.

Outpatient Care

MS. MYDER: As a beneficiary representative, I want to stress my concern about the impacts of Medicare changes that are taking place.

I think you began to talk about these impacts in terms of the skilled nursing facility and that is, the changes that have taken place. Solutions apparently will be discussed as the budget pressure goes away. The question is: will the pressure on Medicare go away?

I think there's enough pressure already. The PPS system has increased or is, I think, shifting costs to the Part B area. That's where beneficiaries pay the highest levels of cost sharing. That's where we all know the pressure on the budget is greatest.

Ms. BURKE: Where in the Part B area are we shifting?

Ms. MYDER: From inpatient to outpatient, for example. Services provided by physicians.

Ms. BURKE: Is that a negative? Are you arguing it's a negative?

Ms. MYDER: I'm saying that attention to reform needs to be placed, probably sooner and in greater amounts than it is already, on factors outside of hospital reimbursement, for example. Any reform in home health payment, or any reform that includes skilled nursing facilities, to encourage these providers to take on sicker patients, I don't think can wait as long as it appears that we will have to wait. That's not just from a beneficiary perspective, but it's from the perspective of caring for people when they leave the hospital.

So what I'm suggesting is that we have a problem to be dealt with now. I think it will be more of a problem and, while I guess we're all saying that we need to give attention to the Part B side and to the nonhospital providers, I think that it should be sooner than you suggest the budgetary constraints would allow.

Ms. BURKE: In fact, Janet, I don't think there's a delay for lack of interest. I think that there is a tremendous desire to understand more clearly what takes place in those institutions.

There is some research under way, for example, the use of RUGs[2] and some of the other kinds of payment changes that attempt to look at resource allocation in long-term care facilities, to try and devise some kind of a reimbursement system. The nursing home industry, as I suggested, is anxious to get away from the current system they

---

[2]Editor's note: Resource utilization groups (RUGs) are experimental patient groupings based on the amount of staff time spent in specific contact with long-term care patients. Research funded by the Health Care Financing Administration and the state of New York is in progress at Rensselaer Polytechnic Institute.

have, as are we, as I think are the individual consumer groups.

The question is: what have we got to replace it with, and does what we have to replace it with make more sense? What you don't want to do is put into place something that runs the risk of discouraging services being provided in those settings. You want to do something that makes it better. A full expansion of cost-based reimbursement isn't going to be the answer the Congress is going to buy off on.

Now the question is what else we have available to us. What do we know about the patients that are cared for in skilled nursing facilities? We know that their average length of stay is "X," but we don't really know, necessarily, about what really takes place in those institutions in terms of the kinds of resources they actually use.

I think our understanding is growing, but we've been less involved with the details of that service in recent years in terms of Medicare than we have on the hospital side. We knew far more about the resources used in an acute care institution.

So I think there's tremendous pressure to try and do something about SNF care and about home care; but I think that there is some hesitancy because we want to put into place something that makes sense, not something that's just a short-term answer that may make the situation worse.

I think you're absolutely correct. We have to do it fast, because there's clearly pressure to get people out of hospitals and into those settings.

Ms. MYDER: And they're already doing that.

Ms. BURKE: That's absolutely right.

MR. SEIDMAN: I think this relates directly to the point that I made, too. That is, if you're considering the question, for example, of the percent paid by the government and you simply project what has been done before or the percent paid by the beneficiary—I don't think anybody is arguing that we should not be transferring some services out of the hospital, but the payment system is such that when you do that you increase the cost paid out of pocket by the beneficiary. We ought to be taking account of that, rather than ignoring it. I think at this point we're ignoring it.

Freedom of Choice

MR. PAULY: Just wanted to ask about a dimension of quality that could be reduced but probably would save substantially on cost, and inquire what Congress' attitude is on that.

That really is the dimension of free choice or access to whatever provider the beneficiary chooses. If the most convenient hospital or the most attractive hospital is the one with a practice pattern that's associated with frequent hospitalizations or use of outpatient care that's expensive as opposed to less expensive physician office practice, is there any disposition to think of a limitation of choice in order to save the taxpayers money along the PPO [preferred provider organization] line?

MS. BURKE: I guess the person who's been most outspoken on that issue is Henry Waxman, who has absolutely no interest in limiting freedom of choice on the Medicaid side. So I can't imagine he would be very interested on the Medicare side.

MR. PAULY: Despite what the states have, in fact, done on it?

MS. BURKE: Despite what the states have done in narrow cases. They've been restricted to a certain extent as to what they could, in fact, do. That was a big fight, to allow that kind of contracting to take place. I think it's still open as to how successful it's been for both the individual beneficiary and for the institutions.

I think that there are risks in both cases. One, in freedom of choice, in locking people in and, in effect, not allowing them to vote with their feet. Also, in terms of their measure of quality—how they respond to an institution may be affected by their ability to choose.

Now your point is that there are institutions that do more admissions—I mean, the re-admission rates—or that use more costly outpatient services. The outpatient side is, no doubt, something that is a concern to us. But on the inpatient side, it has become less of an issue because of the DRG payment model. DRGs attempt to be neutral in the sense that they pay a set amount so that it's not in the institution's best interest to try and load up for that particular service.

I think the risk, again, is that you really want people to be able to make decisions based on what they perceive that their needs are and the people that are caring for them perceive that they need. But there will be those who will argue that the best way to do that is through some kind of a lock-in, the kind of example that the private insurance companies have moved toward through the creation of PPOs.

They give benefits for those going to their providers versus somebody else's. You know, the same concept an HMO uses in terms of a lock-in, in terms of the institutions that they utilize. You pay a penalty if you go outside that system. So I think there is a growing number of individuals who are going into systems that limit their choices. As a result, you may find growing acceptance of that. But I think, in the past, that's been difficult for Medicare to put into place, given the beneficiaries who have, in fact, argued that they want to have that range of choices, that Medicare guaranteed them that range of choices, and that, as long as the payment model doesn't benefit a provider from doing more than they ought to do, then what difference should it make to Medicare? I suspect you're going to see growing acceptance of that concept. Therefore, you may see some willingness to do it for Medicare.

On the Medicaid side, that has been a big issue and it's only been narrow changes in the last couple of years that have expanded the abilities of the states to lock people in for certain kinds of things. But it was with a number of caveats—what you could do to get out and how quickly you could choose.

The states argued that they had to be able to lock in patients for a specific period of time or they couldn't get the providers to be willing to participate. In effect, if you can't guarantee them somebody's going to come there for a month or six months or whatever, it doesn't work. So you have to give us some kind of a control.

Limitations on choice have been the subject of an awful lot of debate. I think there are people who are concerned about it.

Long-Term Care

Ms. YOUNG: All the conversation seems to be about budget limits, but watching Congress one realizes that it's quite responsive to the electoral process. Wouldn't demographics perhaps lead to an opposite pressure, or pressure for expanded nursing home care and this type of thing? Is there going to be any addressing of this as we get an older and older population and more and more people in their eighties more likely needing long-term nursing home care?

Ms. BURKE: Well, I think that's what's behind a push to revisit the Medicare benefit, the structure of the Medicare benefit, because of the aging of the population, because of the number of old, old. But again, you have to realize that you've got a very small percentage of elderly who are institutionalized.

You have a large number of elderly who are not, who might place their priorities somewhere else. Bert Seidman, I think, would probably argue that some of the other things that we don't pay for, including outpatient drugs, those kinds of things, are the bigger concern to a different group. But I think that there is pressure to revisit the benefit.

30

I think nursing home care is an issue that, again, we've avoided, because we're afraid to get into it not knowing what the solution would be. But it forces us to revisit what Medicare was intended to do, which was an acute care benefit, not a long-term care benefit—whether it's willing to trade off acute care for long-term care and, therefore, find some other way of financing long-term care.

I think you're right. The aging of the population will force us to revisit that, without a doubt. But I don't think we yet know what people want the outcome to be. You know, are they willing to trade off one for the other, because it's not going to be that we will simply add "X" dollars. It's going to be what are you willing to give up in order to add, at least in the short term.

Ms. YOUNG: Well, that's the question I had. You have a population in which you have a lot of very old elderly, over 80, a large number of younger elderly but they can see what might be their future, and perhaps an equally large number of people around 50 who are starting to wonder whether or not all their resources are going to pay for the parent who's still alive.

Ms. BURKE: That's right.

Ms. YOUNG: Wouldn't you get a tremendous pressure to do something about nursing home care?

Ms. BURKE: Yes, but I would assume you are also going to get tremendous pressure on the private insurance market to begin to address that, at least I would hope you would, in terms of long-term care insurance.

Ms. YOUNG: Can it be done on the private side?

Ms. BURKE: I don't know the answer to that.

MR. SALISBURY: Jack Kittredge, would you like to comment on that?

MR. KITTREDGE: The answer is no, but—it's a very difficult benefit to design and market on a financially sound basis. As a matter of fact, it really has to be marketed well before there's a need for the coverage to accumulate adequate funds. And it raises some issues as to what cash value, if any, you should have. If you look at it realistically, the cash value should be available only to the ill, not to the well.

I think there are some tax questions involved, because I think there's a real question as to whether or not the reserves accumulated by an insurer can be treated as a deductible reserve for tax purposes. Just

31

a myriad of issues. There have been some very limited experiments so far which haven't proven a great deal.

Home Health Care

MR. SCIOLI: I think that if we were to summarize the history of the delivery of medical care in America, it probably could be stated that today's solutions become tomorrow's problems.

It would seem to me that the most realistic proposal is one which creates reimbursement incentives to provide care at a required level and at the least cost. For many types of services, that includes out-patient care. The cost sharing of that outpatient care, however, may end up discouraging use of those services.

I'm curious to know what the rationale would be, as an example, for stating today that we should have cost-sharing requirements imposed on home health for those types of services that the system is trying to promote. It may result in what has occurred in emergency rooms countrywide, where 50 percent or more of patients are non-emergent. If this is going to drive people into nursing homes or other institutions, then it needs to be rethought.

It seems to me that we also need to think about what kind of care needs to be provided for the treatment of chronic illnesses, because many of those are going to be treatable on an outpatient basis. Yet, the case of a person who has arthritis, for example, could easily become a situation where a family becomes obligated to institutionalize.

I'd like your comments about these, particularly the impact that reimbursement cost sharing might have on the use of outpatient services.

MS. BURKE: Well, the only benefit that doesn't have cost sharing is home health. I mean, it's the only one left in Medicare. Everything else does.

I think the arguments presumably put forth by the administration and those in the past have been, one, equity—that it ought to be treated like all the other services that are covered under the Medicare program; two, there's continuing debate over whether or not cost sharing discourages inappropriate utilization or results in the avoidance of the appropriate level of care, that people avoid going to get care because they're going to have cost sharing and, therefore, get sicker, therefore more costly when they're cared for.

You know, I'm not sure that anybody has the answer to that question. But I think on the home health benefit, it's also been argued in terms of utilization. It's been one of the fastest growing benefits in the program in recent years and whether cost sharing has any deterrent effect in terms of inappropriate utilization. I think that broad range of arguments will be put forward by folks that have suggested cost sharing.

With respect to the nature of the benefit, you are absolutely correct that there are a lot of things that are forcing us—again, going back to the long-term care issue, but just generally—forcing us to reexamine the benefit that Medicare provides.

We are now able to do things on an ambulatory basis that we never even thought possible. I have a very close friend who runs a home health agency in Tennessee who argues that she can basically keep anybody at home, if you give her enough resources to do so. The technology is such that you can now care for really quite ill people at home. So the question is: should Medicare rethink what it thought home health services were designed to provide?

Again, the payment model, the results of the DRGs in pushing people out of institutions, is, in fact, raising questions about what we ought to pay for. I mean questions about infusion therapy, and what, in fact, should you allow to take place in the home setting? What will Medicare recognize?

For a long time, there was concern about letting things take place in the home that were not really appropriately done there and that there was risk to the patient. It's the same thing that we went through when we expanded coverage to include ambulatory surgical centers, the question of what things could appropriately be done in an outpatient setting or on an ambulatory basis that were of a quality that we felt was sufficient for the Medicare beneficiary.

You don't want to set up a system that encourages people to do things that really are not safe. So, we sort of went through that same debate, and we continue to struggle on the ambulatory/surgical side in terms of the expansion of the list and what can, in fact, be done reasonably.

There's both a quality concern about what you're willing to allow to take place and then there's the question of what we can now do that we were not able to do that's forcing us to rethink what we can do on the outpatient side.

I think there's a lot of willingness to expand the outpatient service side to provide incentives for more and more things to be taking place in that setting. But it forces us to rethink what we've paid for in the past and how best to pay for it now.

So you don't again, as you suggest, create a problem that has to be solved next time around. You're right. We create problems every time we fix a problem; they become tomorrow's problems.

The manpower distribution issue is a good example of the best desires in the world in terms of increasing the number of physicians in the community. Now here we are, trying to retrench.

So you're absolutely right. That inevitably happens. So you go along and you try and correct those mistakes. The ESRD program is another good example. I mean, you look at what we did originally with the ESRD program in terms of trying to encourage people to increase access to dialysis and so forth, and then you come to 1978 and realize that all the dialysis basically had moved to an institutional setting. We were paying $25,000 to $30,000 a patient a year for dialysis because we basically discouraged them from dialyzing at home.

So we went back and tried to reshift it so that you had more incentives for people to dialyze at home. Then people complained that we were forcing people to go home who ought not to be home. So they wanted to shift it back. I mean, you're absolutely right. I don't know how to avoid—

MR. SCIOLI: We're also seeing home health visits, the cost of a single skilled-nursing visit, costing more than a day in a nursing home.

MS. BURKE: Yes. And you also have occupational therapy that costs more than skilled nursing on a home health basis. I wonder why, but that's my own bias. But you're right. It does. And the nursing homes will argue that it's cheaper to take care of people in nursing homes, and we would argue that maybe that's not the best place to care for them.

Overutilization

MR. MOSER: Could I shift gears just a second? It occurs to me in analyzing private programs that overutilization is one of our greatest causes of cost increase. I haven't heard a great deal about what's been done under the Medicare programs to perhaps assess for the same kind of problem within the Medicare system.

I guess what I'm thinking about is: I've heard figures that said that 70 percent of the total dollars spent by Medicare were spent in the patient's last year of life. I don't know if that's true or not, but I've seen that figure someplace. If that's the case, has anybody done anything to assess what percentage of these dollars were spent where there was "a reasonable hope" for cure, or whether they were merely spent for easing the pain and suffering of the individual?

Ms. BURKE: Some people know more about that kind of thing than I do. I don't know of anything right off the top of my head. I'm sure there's been something.

Ms. GORNICK: I'm with the Office of Research at the Health Care Financing Administration [HCFA]. First, I'll try to respond to your question with regard to the use of Medicare dollars in the last year of life.

The figure is more like 30 percent, and the study happened to be done in our office. By and large, it did not appear, just from indirect evidence, that there were a whole lot of Medicare expenditures for heroic efforts. For example, analysis of the data shows that the proportion of decedents in 1978 who had expenditures that were greater than $15,000 was relatively small, like 6 percent.

Then I wanted to also make a few comments about the questions that were raised about the impact of PPS on the beneficiaries. I just wanted to point out that HCFA has established a program in which we're going to try to look at a number of issues with regard to the impact of PPS on the beneficiaries. The usual ones will be looking at the differences in admission rates and length-of-stay mortality rates, and postsurgical mortality rates.

The first data for post-PPS will be available this year. But I did want to also point out that I was interested in Bert Seidman's comment about being interested in beneficiary out-of-pocket expenditures. We can definitely look at that. We had planned to look at that. We were going to start by looking just at Part A, but I can promise we'll look at Part B, too, to see what the cost shifting might have been.

Preventive Health Care

Ms. SOMMERS: We should take advantage of the reprieve from an immediate crisis in Medicare funding to go beyond mere tinkering. We now have an opportunity to rethink some of the basic premises on which its current cost-saving provisions are based. It is possible that some of these provisions may be penny-wise but pound-foolish.

For example, if the objective is to reduce unnecessary program expenditures, we cannot assume that deductible and copayment provisions of Part B, designed to reduce use of physician services, are always the answer. They often may be counterproductive. By discouraging beneficiaries from timely access to health services that can reduce risks of future serious illness, they ignore the principle of preventive maintenance, long incorporated into the routine practices of all well-managed industries.

Before Medicare begins to pick up its share of physician bills, beneficiaries must pay $75 up front each year in addition to their Part B premiums. This requirement undoubtedly deters large numbers of asymptomatic people from seeking low-cost tests for colorectal, breast, and cervical cancer, adding to the burden of the very expensive treatments required when such diseases become diagnosed at later stages. In addition, it undoubtedly deters many people with diagnosed hypertension from obtaining the regular physician monitoring they need to avoid medical crises. (The Rand health insurance study demonstrated a significant relationship between deductible provisions and uncontrolled hypertension.) Again, large numbers of expensive, avoidable operations and hospitalizations can result. Among the hospitalizations paid for by Medicare during the first nine months of fiscal year 1985, the DRGs for cardiovascular conditions were by far the most frequently occurring. During this period, the program paid for more than 330,000 such hospital discharges.

Appropriate anticipatory care could also avoid at least some significant proportion of the large numbers of stroke victims and people with diabetes-associated blindness and amputations that eventually require lifelong care in nursing homes. Medicare pays the costs for approximately 22,000 limb amputations among diabetic beneficiaries each year.

The Medicare program's exclusion of preventive services such as influenza immunization from its benefit package should also be reappraised. A task force of the Department of Health and Human Services and the Canadian government is currently developing a list of preventive services of scientifically proven efficacy that it will recommend be offered to people in different age groups at specified intervals of periodicity. It would be unfortunate if changes in the Medicare program do not take advantage of the task force findings and thus be guided by policies that seek to limit improvements in the health status of older people to wise allocations of necessarily limited expenditures.

Impact of Changes in Eligibility

Remarks of Karen Williams

Ms. WILLIAMS: I want to begin my remarks by commending EBRI for its perseverance on behalf of the Medicare beneficiaries. This seminar comes at a time when, as you know, the Medicare solvency problem has just been declared a nonissue. Thanks to the most recent trustees' report, it looks like Congress won't really consider serious reforms until sometime in the early 1990s.

By your participation here today I know that you believe, as I do, that the crisis in Medicare financing is far from over. Although the trust fund may be solvent through 1998 if the economy holds up, there's still no better time than the present to look at reforms that would sustain solvency over a longer period of time. In order for incremental reforms to really be adequate, they have to be allowed a maximum amount of time to take effect. This is true whether you're talking payment reform, benefit restructuring, or beneficiary cost sharing. Only through the cumulative effects of small changes can we hope to avoid a major upheaval in this entitlement program.

I've agreed to discuss the impact of proposed changes in Medicare eligibility, but I want to add my institutional disclaimer to those made by other speakers. My participation in this seminar is not for the purpose of furthering HIAA's [Health Insurance Association of America] position or views. I am simply here to broaden the debate on solvency. To accomplish that, I'm going to raise a series of questions that I think ought to be answered before we go ahead with eligibility changes. I will then pull together data from a variety of sources to try to answer those questions.

I'm going to presume, as the other speakers have, that you folks are basically familiar with the eligibility proposals and the basic structure of Medicare eligibility. If not, there's a little brochure in your package that will help you, or you can ask your neighbor. I'll understand.

Working-Aged Provisions

I'm going to begin by dismissing several of the small-ticket items that you've heard of so far this morning, starting with the working-aged proposals.

The working-aged provisions and other similar statutory attempts to make private coverage primary were supposed to save about $650 million annually. Despite a slow start, HCFA now estimates they've netted about $450 million.

As private carriers, our industry is trying to work more closely with Medicare to better coordinate the implementation of those provisions. Therefore actual savings ought to increase in the near future.

There's one more change for the working aged that is currently being proposed by the administration. They would extend such provisions to those active workers older than 69. The proposal would save an additional $120 million if it were fully implemented.

Past and proposed ideas for making Medicare coverage secondary to private coverage total $770 million. Only in the context of the trust fund deficit would you think of three-quarters of a billion dollars as being a small amount. Given the crisis that we're facing, I would say that this is still a relatively small-ticket item and warrants no further discussion at this point.

Approaches to Means Testing

Means testing has come up in several contexts. In a sense, it does not relate to eligibility, but I'll describe several approaches to means testing, and state why I'm dismissing each of them.

I think means testing of eligibility per se, that is, denial of all Medicare benefits to new retirees unless they contribute more money, is a politically unworkable proposal. As several other speakers have mentioned, this would change the program into more of a welfare concept. Since most workers have contributed to Medicare over their working lifetime, they feel that their eligibility ought not to be jeopardized by their postretirement income. Therefore, this kind of change should be considered as a proposal of absolute last resort. For that reason, I'm not going to spend more time on it.

Means testing of Part B premiums is probably administrable if it's linked very closely to tax liability and tax collection. But I would propose to you that, if the Part B premium that results from means testing were high enough to have significant savings, it would probably be high enough to encourage people to bail out of Part B coverage and into the supplemental market.

Some have suggested means testing of cost sharing, that is, to vary coinsurance and deductibles by the level of postretirement income. We've talked about this in our industry, and John Troy could probably add something to this discussion, if he would like. It seems to us that that would be very difficult to administer.

There is a third option that I don't think has really been proposed, but I'm sure it's one that will be considered. That option is, in effect, the taxation of Medicare benefits. It's conceivable that one could impute the actuarial value of Medicare benefits received and add that to the taxable income of the elderly. Although this idea may be administratively feasible, I suggest to you that it runs into many of the arguments that are currently levied against the taxation of employee benefits such as the real value of imputed income. I will not divert our seminar today by discussing the taxation of employee benefits.

Medicare Eligibility

That leaves us with delays in eligibility. Two proposals for delay have been suggested so far. The first proposal would delay eligibility for one month. Instead of becoming eligible for Medicare in the month in which you turn 65, you become eligible at the beginning of the following month. That proposal has been considered for several years in a row. The annual savings estimate is $180 million. Again, this is not significant in terms of the trust fund deficit.

The more significant proposal and the one on which I will spend the bulk of my time would delay Medicare eligibility for two years. Rather than age 65, the age of eligibility would gradually increase until no one becomes eligible for Medicare until the age of 67.

I'll confess to you that, when I got to this point in thinking through my presentation, I grew bored. It seemed to me that a two-year delay was the only eligibility proposal worth further analysis, and, frankly, I presumed that I could guess the results. I assumed that Medicare's two-year delay corresponded with the recently enacted two-year delay in Social Security. I figured most employees were currently retiring at 65. I also figured that, for the half or less who retire early, their employers were continuing group coverage for some of these people. Finally, I assumed that the majority of early retirees could get private policies at quite reasonable rates relative to their Social Security income.

Well, I was wrong on all counts. So, if you made these same assumptions and began to daydream at the beginning of this presentation, I would encourage you to revive your interest because you're likely to find the remainder of my remarks rather unsettling.

Frankly, I was startled by what I learned about coverage for early retirees and shocked by how much I could not find out about their coverage. I'm going to describe for you existing early retirement trends and employer coverage for early retirees, now and in the future. I will also describe retiree income and estimate the cost of individual policies.

Trends in Retirement and Coverage

For starters, the Social Security Administration [SSA] now has a law which delays Social Security benefits for two years. You would expect the Medicare delay to parallel the Social Security delay. It does not. They are 25 years out of sync.

The Social Security delay does not begin until the year 2000. It increases age of eligibility by two months each year until the year 2012. Starting in the year 2017, the age of eligibility again increases by two months per year. The two-year delay isn't fully phased in until the year 2022, 22 years after it began. The Social Security Advisory Council suggested phasing in the Medicare delay over six years, commencing in 1985 and ending in 1991.

The other difference between the Medicare delay and the Social Security delay is that, under Medicare, the retiree would not receive any Medicare benefits until reaching the new age of eligibility. Under the Social Security delay, a retiree would still be eligible for reduced benefits at age 62. In the worst case, the benefits received would be reduced further than they currently are. Currently, a retiree at age 62 receives 80 percent of full benefits. After the Social Security delay is fully phased in, a 62-year-old retiree would receive 70 percent of full benefits.

In my view, a Medicare delay of two years really means retiring before full Social Security benefits are available and before any Medicare coverage is available. It is logical to ask, who now retires before Medicare benefits are available and what are their coverage options?

According to Social Security actuaries approximately 80 percent of all eligible males begin collecting Social Security benefits before age 63. Fifteen percent of those men are on the disability rolls. Sixty-five percent have opted for early retirement and reduced benefits. The percentage of the eligible population receiving Social Security benefits was greater than 80 percent for elderly women.

Are these folks healthy enough to risk going without coverage or are they getting coverage someplace else?

SSA has recently published a series of bulletins about the health of the elderly. Please bear in mind that there is quite a bit of argument about the survey instruments used and whether people ever accurately report either their health status or their income. The latest SSA survey looked at 65-year-olds first receiving Social Security benefits in 1982. Two-thirds of all beneficiaries reported no health conditions that would result in a work limitation. If self-assessment is accurate, new retirees are a relatively healthy group.

To answer whether retirees are getting coverage elsewhere, Deborah Chollet of EBRI and I tried to weave together various data sources. Although we were frustrated by lack of uniform data elements, we reached some tentative conclusions that are the best that we can do today.

First, approximately half of all workers are employed in firms with less than 100 employees. Three out of four such firms do not provide health care coverage for early retirees. For the other half of all workers, those in larger firms, one out of three have no early retiree health coverage. If you relate these statistics arithmetically, you'll find that a little over 50 percent of all workers who retire early do so without employer-sponsored health benefits.

I then asked whether employers who provide retiree benefits have an incentive to continue providing such coverage. I learned that, in fact, there are growing *disincentives* to providing retiree coverage.

Two recent court cases appear to limit employers' ability to control their liability for retirees' benefits. In the Bethlehem Steel case, the court ruled that the employer could not reduce health benefits to its retirees even though it was reducing benefits to its active workers through the adoption of higher coinsurance and deductibles, pre-admission screening, and the like. In another case, the White Farm Equipment Company, in anticipation of bankruptcy, tried to terminate its retirement coverage by offering retirees the option of converting their policy or reallocating available funds to some other plan. The court ruled that the company could not terminate its liability.

Recent changes under DEFRA could provide disincentives to retiree coverage. One such change is that the reserves placed in trust for retiree medical costs appear to be taxable. Deductions for employer contributions beyond those based on *current* medical liability may not be allowable deductions. This change is particularly critical since the cost of retiree health care can be expected to increase faster than the cost of active-worker benefits. DEFRA also establishes a 100-percent penalty tax. An employer who prefunds his retirement benefits, but overfunds based on what is actually needed in the future, may lose access to the additional funds that he set aside.

Perhaps the greatest disincentive is that health care costs are increasing faster for retirees than for active workers. AT&T recently estimated that from 1970 through 1984 its annual increase in medical expense plan costs for active workers was 16.8 percent, yet overall

41

those costs increased 18.2 percent per year, reflecting a higher rate of increase in retiree health care costs. Among covered retirees, early retirees are significantly more costly to insure than retirees over the age of 65. AT&T estimated their cost for an over-65 retiree at about $400 a year, and their cost for an under-65 retiree at $1,500 a year.

If you think about that in terms of working-aged proposals, to the extent we finally are able to implement them, and the shift that you've heard about from Part B under Medicare, that same shift will increase Medicare supplement costs. So, for employers providing health care coverage to their retirees, that coverage will become more expensive.

Individual Coverage Options

What are the opportunities for individual coverage? Some employers offer conversion policies for early retirees and their dependents. Such provisions allow a retiree or dependent to obtain an individual policy without regard to pre-existing conditions and without a waiting period before benefits are payable. Although the conversion option is, of course, desirable, it is typically used by those retirees and dependents who, in fact, have pre-existing conditions. Therefore, adverse selection drives up the cost of conversion policies.

I have to put a big caveat around the numbers I'm going to give you now, because they are in no way statistically reliable. We did a little phone survey on the price of individual policies for those aged 60 to 64 with and without pre-existing conditions. We found that coverage under conversion policies is approximately $220 a month for an individual aged 60 to 64. There was a differential of a few dollars between the sexes. By comparison, premiums are about $140 a month for individual policies with fairly standard coverage for someone aged 60 to 64 with no pre-existing conditions. The elderly in this age category would obviously opt for individual insurance, if they don't have pre-existing conditions.

Given the expense of monthly premiums, the question naturally arises as to whether the financial resources of early retirees are sufficient to permit purchase of individual insurance. Deborah Chollet and I tried to determine how many early retirees have individual coverage. We are as yet unable to do so. While failing to obtain actual figures, we can compare these annual premium costs to typical Social Security income.

In 1983 the average monthly Social Security benefit for a retired worker with full benefits was $441. For the spouse it was $226. That's a total income per couple of $667. Since we're looking here at early retirees who may receive only 80 percent of their full benefit, the monthly benefit for a couple is reduced to $534.

Total private individual premiums for this couple, if neither one had pre-existing conditions, would be $280 per month, or more than 50 percent of their Social Security check. If both had pre-existing conditions and used a conversion option from an employer, the combined premiums would total $440 per month, or more than 75 percent of their Social Security benefit. While this is a significant burden to those elderly relying only on Social Security benefits, the elderly are not a homogeneous group with regard to income and assets. Therefore, it is still very difficult to draw conclusions about how many early retirees could not afford private insurance coverage.

The Elderly's Financial Resources

The recent Economic Report of the President contains these insights into the total financial resources of the elderly. The report estimates that Social Security benefits represent only 40 percent of all elderly income. The balance comes 25 percent from income related to assets, 15 percent from earnings, 15 percent from pensions, and the remainder from public assistance and family assistance. The report says that the percentage of all elderly living below the poverty line is now 14 percent. This is lower than the 15-percent rate for nonelderly poor. However, the poor elderly are another nonhomogeneous group.

In 1983, the poverty line was $393 per month for elderly individuals living alone, and most elderly do live alone. Twenty-six percent of all the elderly living alone in their own households fall below the poverty line. Elders with spouses were financially better off. Only 9 percent of those fell below the poverty line.

Private-sector pension plans and retiree health benefits correlate with postretirement income levels. If you have sufficient total retirement income to purchase individual health insurance during early retirement, you are also more likely to already have some kind of insurance through your employer. If you don't have employer health coverage, you are far less likely to have the postretirement income to purchase it.

In summary, the delay of entitlement to age 67 is the only Medicare eligibility change proposed so far that has sufficient savings, administrative feasibility, and some political viability. However, the current proposal for a six-year transition is totally out of step with the recently enacted delay in Social Security benefits. Yet, 80 to 90 percent of the elderly already retire before they become eligible for Medicare benefits.

We do not have good information on how current early retirees pay for their health care. We know that, for the majority, employer coverage is not available, and much of what is available reflects conversion policies that are expensive. You can expect to see a reduction in employer-based retiree health benefits for several reasons, including changes in the tax code, recent court decisions, and the increasing cost of retiree health care.

In short, a delay to age 67 would disenfranchise about two million elderly per year, at a time when employer benefits are less likely to be available for early retirees and while the private market may have become too expensive for many.[1]

---

[1]Author's note: My presentation focused on the extent of employer-based group coverage. There are other potential sources of group coverage which were not discussed. These include: a) employer-based coverage for retired workers with part-time jobs; b) retired workers covered by working spouses; and c) group coverage made available to members of professional or social organizations.

The Impact of Medicare Financing Reforms: A View From the Private Sector

Paper by John F. Troy

Introduction

This forum is intended to review Medicare financing reforms and their possible impact on the private sector. My role is to give an outside perspective on the program and future financing options, particularly as seen from the private sector. I will be reflecting my own opinions, as well as facts that I have gathered or synthesized from others. I am not speaking for the insurance industry, although having spent most of my life in that industry, I am clearly influenced by it. This paper will distill much of my own thinking about these matters, after working for a number of years on health financing, and Medicare intermediary issues, and serving on task forces addressing Medicare trust fund solvency and benefit redesign questions.

Let me state a few assumptions or beliefs at the beginning. First, we need to keep Medicare as a social insurance program available to all elderly Americans. There are several reasons for this belief, including the importance of the historic social contract that promised insurance coverage for all elderly in return for working-life contributions of payroll taxes into the hospital insurance (HI) fund. In addition, changes in universality of coverage would institutionalize two types or two "classes" of health care. While some might argue that we already have several types or classes of care, which I would agree with, we still have a single basic program for all people over 65 (and the disabled) that ensures a very good floor of coverage, at least for acute care. All citizens can participate in Medicare without going through a public assistance-type screening process.

The current Medicare program is quite different, in my mind, from a program such as Medicaid, which is for those whose incomes are below a certain level. If Medicare were "means tested for eligibility," as it is called in the trade, it might quickly become another welfare-type program. If we choose to head in that direction, which might be desirable over the very long haul, an equally long phase-in period would be needed. However, I have seen no outline yet developed for a means-tested Medicare program that would assure adequate health benefits for the elderly, particularly the very old, when heavy expenses are greatest. If we move in that direction, we must develop programs to ensure the availability of private coverage. This would be particularly critical for the very old.

Second, if we are to maintain Medicare for all elderly and disabled Americans, we have reasons for being concerned about Medicare's future. These are well known, certainly to this audience. But a few facts, plus Figure 1 from the new trust fund report [see Appendix C], bear repeating in case anyone thinks that problems of increasing health expenses for the elderly are solved. The drain on the trust fund is because of ever-growing health care costs, although hospital admissions have dropped in recent months and the rate of inflation has slowed. Medicare also pays for increases in the intensity of services, as well as expanding numbers of elderly, especially the so-called "old elderly" (75 + and 85 +). Even with slower rates of growth in unit costs, the proportion of the GNP that will go to health care could climb to 14 percent in the future.[1]

Last year, Americans spent $384.3 billion for health care, an 8.1-percent increase over 1983 (a number that is considered "good news" by most observers). Put another way, the U.S. spent $1,500 per person for health care while Germany, France, Japan, and Great Britain spent $900, $800, $500, and $400, respectively. This disparity raises questions of international competitiveness of American goods and services. While the U.S. rate of increase has clearly slowed and is continuing to look promising, new projections for the future "continue to look dreadful," as Dr. David Rogers, head of the prestigious Robert Wood Johnson Foundation, recently reported. He also said that the nation's health spending will reach $690 billion in 1990 and $1.9 *trillion* in the year 2000[2] (figure 1).

Under current law, receipts and beneficiary contributions will be unable to keep pace with those expenditures, creating a trust fund deficit. The only dispute might be *when* the deficit begins, not *if* it will begin. We should certainly plan now to ensure that the greatest number of options are available to us and we are not forced to act precipitately.

Third, while we have seen some important changes in recent years, benefit design in Medicare continues to encourage the use of more expensive forms of care, while leaving some significant and increasingly important areas uncovered, such as chronic care, nursing home

---

[1] David Rogers, *Annual Report* (Princeton: Robert Wood Johnson Foundation, 1984).
[2] Ibid.

FIGURE 1

Forecasted Health Spending, 1984–2000 (Preliminary Estimates)

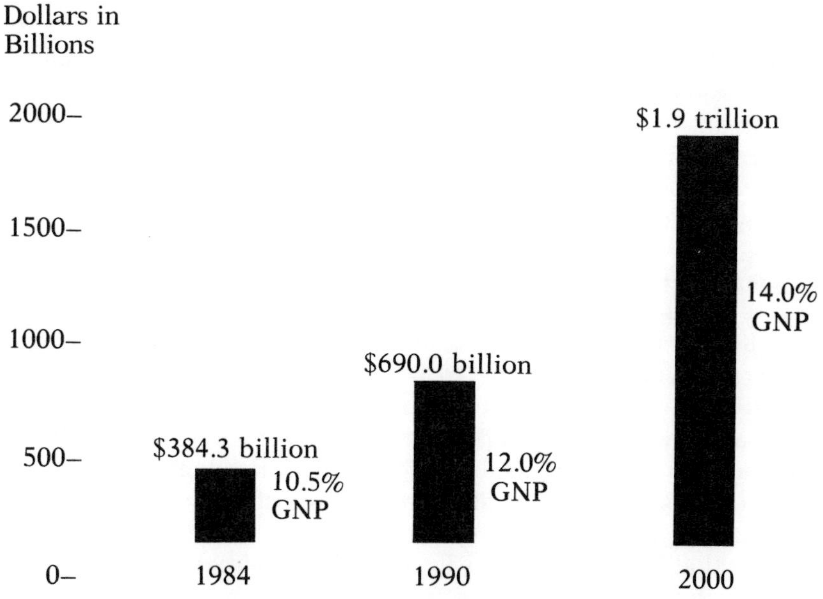

Dollars in
Billions

Source: The Robert Wood Johnson Foundation

care, and patient medications. When reviewing options for change, we should not completely ignore the need to make some fundamental design changes that will more fully reflect the shifts in demography and health-care delivery systems than the system designed 20 years ago when Medicare started. I am not suggesting expansions in coverage, which I am sure would be politically difficult and probably also a policy mistake; I am suggesting that we should re-examine what Medicare pays for now and substitute other services, as we have begun to see as so effective in the substitution of outpatient surgery (e.g., eye surgery) for costlier inpatient surgery. We must also consider new ways to encourage individuals to insure themselves for the other services (e.g., long-term care) to keep pressure off the government to fund public programs for people who have the means over a working career to take care of themselves, if they plan carefully. We are beginning to see again, I believe, a growing national consensus on the issue of individual responsibility for planning for retirement and associated end-of-life costs.

These changes are complicated by the new era of competition. Currently, "competition" is the byword in health care financing and

47

delivery, but the health system is, I believe, a unique arena for competition in this country. We need to have a form of competition which contributes to the societal goal of fair access to quality care for all Americans.

If we are to devise sensible solutions that will work and benefit everyone to the extent possible, then alternative financing arrangements must be examined with providers, beneficiaries, and taxpayers in mind, not just one part of the equation. The balance of this paper is organized from each of their perspectives.

Providers

Hospitals—The recent revolution in the way Medicare pays hospitals is well known to this audience. It is already clear that we are seeing both cost cutting and cost shifting. Insurers certainly welcome the former, while continuing to be harmed by the latter. But the reductions in expenditure growth in hospitals are real, and for now we are all benefitting. In my judgment, we are seeing the results of a confluence of forces: centralized government-fixed pricing for Medicare; business and insurers standing up to hospitals and saying "no more"; and the effects of a myriad of programs and technological advances that have made many formerly hospital-based surgical procedures into routine outpatient services.

All of these factors are having an effect but more is needed. If some proportions of hospitals in crowded urban areas could be closed so the hospitals left would be used most effectively, I believe we would see even more significant economies and further pressure would be removed from the trust fund. Beyond that, we need to make serious efforts to assure that we are paying only for appropriate and effective care. Once the system is much leaner and care is limited to necessary, appropriate, and effective care, the unit costs for hospitals should be fairly reimbursed. Otherwise, in time we could begin to seriously impair quality of care and limit access. Also, as we move toward a more competitive system, we need to be certain that the costs of uncompensated care, graduate medical education, and research are spread proportionately across all payers to ensure a level playing field for all payers and all providers.

Some of the impetus for more arbitrary freezing comes from the belief that there are still considerable inefficiencies, excess capacity, and unnecessary utilization, but once those pockets of inefficiencies are eliminated, the fairness of the unit rates will become critical. If not, we would once again exacerbate the cost-shifting problem. I

48

would hate to see any of those negative effects, but I think we have a way to go before we hit muscle in cutting out the fat in the health system.

At the same time, to help ensure that valuable, new technology is made available to help retire less effective or ineffective technology, I would recommend the creation of a strong advisory committee on technology, with representatives from the affected industries and professions and third-party payers. The committee would advise third-party payers, Congress, and others who might be interested in knowing what technology they should pay for and what might be left out of third-party coverage.

In the interim, there is a great deal to be done to strengthen and expand requirements concerning: (a) pre-admission certification, (b) second opinions for designated surgical procedures, (c) ambulatory surgery for certain procedures, and (d) limiting reimbursement for low-volume/high-cost technology and procedures to certain locations. Each of these steps may be as valuable to ensure excellent quality care as they have potential for total cost savings. The irritating and inconveniencing elements of implementing such programs can be eliminated through public education and dissemination of information on efficacy of treatment, quality, and price.

Physicians—As noted above, I believe that we should get to a stage where we pay an appropriate and fair price for appropriate, effective care. This will be a difficult task. Right now Congress, through Medicare (and Medicaid, for that matter), has simply frozen the fees that the government pays physicians. This approach slows unit-cost inflation and reduces outlays, but does not deal with inequities of the existing system and provides incentives for physicians to recoup their costs by increasing the number of services given.

The growing excess supply of doctors, which could be a serious long-term cost problem, and the clever idea of making it more attractive to be participating physicians seem to be keeping physicians from dropping out of Medicare. Even at fixed prices, lower than wanted, Medicare is a necessary source of revenue and patients, particularly to the younger, debt-burdened physicians in metropolitan areas.

In time, Medicare will have to use other methods of reimbursing physicians. Some surgical procedures lend themselves to bundling of services. Many already have flat or global fees that include pre- and postoperative visits, and the operation itself. These should be systematized and more widely used. Other visits and procedures might use fee schedules.

The key to controlling physician costs by Medicare, as with hos-

49

pitals, will be to change the economic incentives. Consistent with the pluralism that Americans enjoy, there should be many different approaches. The more individuals we have participating in care and/or coverage packages or utilization review programs that modify or reverse some of the current economic incentives, the better. Until then, the growth in the supply of physicians could drive overall health care costs to disturbing heights, even as we see real price discounting and competition among physicians driving down unit costs in some places.

Beneficiaries

Part A (HI) Options—While the suggestions made above would help to hold down the growth of Medicare outlays, which is essential, new revenues are also needed to bring fiscal health to the trust fund in the future. Changes that take more money out of anyone's pockets will always be unpopular, but there is no question that new revenues must be found.

There are a number of financing options that would require Medicare beneficiaries to contribute more. One way would be to add a premium for Part A. It could be (a) a flat premium, (b) graduated according to income, (c) handled through the Medicare program, or (d) handled through the tax system. For example, Davis and Rowland have proposed a system in which financing for Part A (HI) and Part B (SMI) would be merged.[3] A combined premium would be paid from general tax revenues. In turn, the premium level charges would be related to income and administered through the tax system. This could be done any one of several ways, including: (a) a fixed-dollar premium with the poor exempted, (b) a premium set at a constant percentage of adjusted gross income, (c) a premium set at a constant percentage of taxable income, and (d) a premium set at a constant percentage of tax liability.

According to survey research published by Cambridge Reports, Inc., the public seems to favor Medicare reform measures that would require higher-income elderly people to pay an income tax on some value (e.g., one-half of their Medicare benefits). Certainly there is credible experience already with taxing Social Security benefits that suggests a possible national acceptance of this approach.

More Beneficiary Cost Sharing on Combined Options—There are, of course, other, more direct ways to get beneficiaries to pay for the

---

[3] Karen Davis and Diane Rowland, "Medicare Financing Reforms: A New Medicare Premium." *Proceedings of the Conference on the Future of Medicare*, February 1, 1984.

program. As part of our investigation of alternative sources of financing, I asked Travelers actuaries to estimate what the premiums would have to be if federal outlays were allowed to grow only at specified rates. In making these estimates, we assumed that the public wanted to keep a viable Medicare program and thereby would be willing to share more of its costs.

The goal of Travelers research was to determine whether increased cost sharing under certain circumstances was feasible and what the costs would be. The following assumptions were made for the analysis:

- The source of the HI outlays and income is Alternative II-A of the 1985 Annual Report of the Medicare Board of Trustees. Under this alternative, the trust fund will be completely exhausted in the late 1990s.

- The figures for SMI disbursements and income are taken from Alternative II-A of the Annual Report for the years 1985–1987. After 1987, the SMI growth rate was projected to be 10 percent each year. SMI income consists of 75 percent general revenue contributions and 25 percent enrollee premiums and interest income.

- Inflation is set at 5 percent.

- The number of enrollees was projected to grow by slightly over 2 percent per year.

- The payroll tax percentage is held constant and payroll tax base increases are limited to an average wage increase.

- General revenue contributions are held to the 1983 level ($14.9 billion) with increases adjusted only for inflation and the number of enrollees.

- The monthly premium is set to include the SMI income from enrollees (25 percent of program costs) plus the amount needed to cover shortfalls in the HI fund, SMI, or both.

Findings—The results of our research indicate that passing the *total* amount of increased costs on to enrollees would be very difficult. Using the trustees' projections and a 10-percent SMI program growth rate, the total monthly premium (in nominal dollars) rises from $15.50 in 1985 to $22.52 in 1990. This moderate increase through 1990 is possible because surpluses in the HI fund offset those amounts required by the SMI program over and above enrollee contributions and capped general revenues.

After 1990, however, premiums have to rise rapidly to cover shortfalls in both the HI fund and SMI program. As a result, premiums jump to $40.54 in 1992, double by 1995 at $80.53 per month, and more than double again, to $168.01, by 2000. This means that premium levels, in nominal dollars, would increase 45 percent by 1990, 420 percent over the next decade, and 984 percent by 2000. Adjusting the premium levels to 1983 dollars still means that by 1995 the premium would increase by 218 percent to $45.45 and would reach $74.29 in 2000, representing an overall increase of 420 percent. The impact of projected premiums for 1995 on incomes of the elderly is shown in figure 2.

I want to stress that these projections must be considered very rough estimates, as projecting costs of medical care for any appreciable time is very difficult. These figures seem to show, however, that increasing enrollee cost sharing to control federal outlays would look somewhat acceptable for the short term, but the rising costs of medical care and aging of the population raises serious questions as to this approach as a sole strategy for the long term.

Increased enrollee cost sharing under this scenario raises several other important concerns. First, it may not be feasible to limit payroll taxes to current levels and increase general revenue contributions according to the population and inflation. Even if these caps could be implemented, they may force so much enrollee cost sharing that the Medicare program could not survive. Adverse selection will definitely become a consideration at high levels of cost sharing. A cap on Medicare costs may not be feasible in view of the aging of the population, the types of medical services offered, and further technological advances.

Second, if the disparity between program revenues and outlays became too great and cost sharing too burdensome, more people

FIGURE 2
Impact of Projected Premiums on Incomes of the Elderly
(1983 Dollars)

Projected Cash Income of Elderly Families at Age 65	Distribution of Families at Income Levels in 1995	1995 Premium Based on 1985 Trustees' Projections & 10% SMI Growth Rate		Annual Premium as a Percentage of Projected Income in 1995
		Monthly	Annual	
Less than $5,966	21%	$45.45	$545.40	9% of income
$ 5,966 to $11,932	26%	45.45	545.40	9%–5%
$11,933 to $17,898	19%	45.45	545.40	5%–3%
$17,899 to $29,831	19%	45.45	545.40	3%–2%
$29,832 and over	16%	45.45	545.40	2%

March 1985

could qualify for state aid programs. By shifting more costs to people who had been considered "near poor," a new class of people eligible for state aid would be created. States may not be willing or financially able to accommodate increasing numbers of people needing assistance. In addition, state aid programs are funded partially by federal general revenues. If state programs are forced to expand, more general revenues would have to be contributed. It could be difficult to control the growth of costs and general revenues in state aid programs.

Finally, the degree of increased cost sharing would determine its political acceptability. If cost sharing became extreme, as our projections indicate it could, it is likely that there would be substantial opposition from current and future enrollees as well as state governments. Congress would also want to consider whether mandatory participation in Medicare should be imposed. As the level of cost sharing rises, people who cannot or will not pay the increased rates would argue that they should be permitted to opt out of Medicare.

On the other hand, there is a positive aspect to cost sharing. Enrollees who are financially able would be sharing in more of the costs of their health care. Premiums, deductibles, or copayments could be effectively structured to provide maximum financing and incentives for prudent use of services. For this reason, increased cost sharing should be considered in conjunction with other control measures rather than as the single solution to Medicare's problems.

Part B (SMI) Options—There are also specific methods for increasing revenues to Part B that need to be considered. The Congressional Budget Office estimated that if the Part B premium were set at 35 percent of program benefits beginning January 1, 1986, there would be savings of $1.7 billion in the first year (FY86) and $17.2 billion over the five-year period. There are variations on this idea, but the advantages and disadvantages are similar to those discussed above.

The tax system could be used to impose a supplementary income-related premium for physician services. The Part B premium is currently set at 25 percent of program costs. Revenues for the rest of the program's costs come from general revenues. Instead of an across-the-board premium increase, higher-income beneficiaries could pay a supplement as part of their income tax. For example, a 1-percent tax could be imposed on enrollees' taxable income. Rough estimates are that $0.1 billion would be added in 1986 and $2.1 billion over five years (CBO, 1985). An alternative explored by a White House policy group would increase the percentage of program costs paid by individuals with higher incomes. We have no figures on this, but a

53

tax on income could be calculated to produce revenues to cover the imputed value of 50 percent of program costs.

Increasing the Part B deductible from $75 to $200 on January 1, 1986, and indexing it to the CPI would save $610 million in FY86 and $6 billion over a five-year period. While the increase would be costly to some, the deductible started at $50 in 1966, so it has actually remained very low relative to income and benefits since then.

In any given year, about 35 percent of beneficiaries do not present claims that exceed the deductible. With a deductible increase, this percentage clearly would increase, reducing claims costs. Beneficiaries would become more prudent shoppers. At the same time, HMOs and other comprehensive plans that cover everything would become even more attractive.

Another alternative receiving attention is one that moves Medicare into the private sector through a voucher program. Under a voucher system, a fixed-amount voucher would be issued by the government to each Medicare beneficiary, who would then use the voucher to purchase a health benefit plan from a private-sector insurance carrier. While the voucher concept may be appealing, there are several looming concerns that would impact its viability. For example, vouchers must be designed to reflect basic insurance principles and, therefore, must take into account factors such as age, location, and health status. It would appear that participation in a voucher program must be mandatory in order to avoid adverse selection. This is a subject which is very large in scope and will require full study before implementation.

Other Revisions Affecting Parts A and B—There are several other ways to improve the financial outlook for Medicare, but I will only list them since others are covering them in depth. Those options include: (a) delaying eligibility for Parts A and B to the first day of the month following the individual's 65th birthday (estimated savings are $300 million) and (b) advancing the age of eligibility to age 67, phased in at one month per year until 2027.

I would simply note in passing that each of these changes, whether desirable or not for other reasons—and I believe they are, on balance—has important effects on business and industry, since they will end up covering many of the costs. Moreover, state and local governments and other programs (e.g., veterans', disability insurance) become alternative (i.e., other than employer) sources of support for care or coverage until Medicare takes over so that costs of care remain publicly financed, just out of different channels. I do not believe we should make such changes without a full airing of the implications and costs of such changes, giving business and industry opportunities to have their say and make suggestions for improvement in design or phasing. There is a question as to how long the employer community will remain relatively silent while Medicare costs are shifted to it, both directly and indirectly.

Taxpayers

The final perspective is that of the taxpayers. A proposal often considered is to *increase payroll taxes*. It is difficult to defend this approach since there is such strong feeling in the corporate community that an increase in the payroll tax would be very burdensome to employers, further disadvantaging U.S. employers in terms of international markets. Also, during recessions, high labor costs aggravate unemployment and may slow recovery.

But a payroll tax increase of, for example, 0.1 percent (.05 for employees and .05 for employers), according to a recent Congressional Budget Office report, would generate approximately $99 billion over the 1986–1990 period. Thus, not only is it administratively simple, it raises a lot of money. Also, such a broad-based tax is most like an insurance premium which is spread across a large population and paid when people are healthy. But payroll taxes are regressive, fall heavily on two-earner couples, and add to labor costs. It is a tough call, but I have become convinced that, given the nature of the Medicare program, the payroll tax remains a very logical source of funding. In this connection, if our goal is to maintain a viable program, the program should cover all employees of state and local governments, including the four million not now covered.

In general, I am opposed to solving the HI trust fund problem by drawing on *general revenues* or increasing the amount of general revenues that go into SMI. The already crisis proportion of the federal deficit suggests that no more direct demands on general revenues are needed, although the income tax is more progressive and a broader-based tax than many others. But the traditional argument that general revenue-financed programs are less controllable and an invitation to profligacy are simply no longer true. If anything, the opposite is the case. No less than the president has said that Social Security does not need to be pared down because it has its own fiscally sound trust fund.

A comparatively simple way to gain general revenues would be to add a percent surcharge to the income tax due, earmarked for Medicare. This would obviously be a way to bring almost everyone into

55

the system who has a certain level of income. It would spread the costs out over a lifetime and include in the Medicare supplement tax income from nonpayroll sources.

Excise Taxes on Alcohol and Tobacco—One proposal with sufficient surface appeal to have been supported by the Social Security Advisory Council suggested that additional taxes on tobacco and alcohol would be levied and earmarked for Medicare. "Sin taxes" are always popular, but they are administratively and politically more complicated than meets the eye. The revenue bases for these taxes are large but generally these federal taxes have not been raised much over the years. They are also regressive. While smoking is clearly dangerous to an individual's health, the empirical evidence to support an argument related to financing Medicare on both sides is weak.

Interfund Borrowing—This is not really a solution to the Medicare problem. It may help buy time and it allows policymakers to think the problem is less critical than it is, but, in the end, sufficient funds to pay for commitments are needed.

Tax Cap—A tax on employer contributions to employee health plans or a cap on the amount of tax-free employee health benefits with revenues dedicated to Medicare seems like a very bad idea to me, and it is clearly opposed by the insurance industry, as well as labor unions, senior citizen groups, and many health professional organizations. First, it increases the burden on employers when they do not need more such costs. Second, the millions of workers who enjoy employer health insurance should be encouraged to insure themselves, not discouraged. A tax break to encourage health insurance purchasing is, to me, a good example of policy that, on balance, serves the public interest. Our research indicates that with a mature health tax cap, millions of workers would drop out of plans, damaging the viability of plans, and increasing the amount of uncompensated care. The recently discussed "floor" or inclusion in employees' taxable income of the first $x of employer contributions to health benefits is an interesting variation of the tax cap. At low levels it would avoid some of the difficulties of the cap, particularly that dealing with inequitable treatment of workers and adverse selection. However, it is probably a more regressive approach and less politically appealing.

Employment-based health plans are a major resource of this country and tax changes which threaten the strength of these plans would, I believe, be contrary to the public interest.

Currently there is a limit on the wage or salary base that is used for Social Security taxes. A relative increase in the wage base so that higher-income workers paid more than lower-wage workers would

56

augment the revenues and be considerably more progressive than some of the other options.

Conclusions

I have reviewed a number of financing options for strengthening the fiscal health of Medicare. Recent good news on Medicare's outlook has certainly had a dramatic impact on the political climate for Medicare reform. But I hope we do not all give in to the temptation to wait until the next crisis to craft changes in the Medicare program and that we use this breathing room to develop policy alternatives that will serve the public interest. On that broader note, I would just like to add my concern that a major health-financing problem, exacerbated sharply by what Medicare is doing, has not been properly addressed in this country—that is, uncompensated care. I recognize that that would probably be considered a subject for another meeting and no one likes to see such a broad-issue conference broadened even further. But uncompensated care is a growing problem in this country and the main reason it is growing now is that Medicare and Medicaid and some other payers are paying less proportionately for their patients and, additionally, not sharing the costs of care for others without coverage (i.e., no more cross-subsidization). Something must be done about this national problem. The impact of this problem and its hidden and very uneven effects on the private sector need to be examined and solutions found.

Remarks of John F. Troy

MR. TROY: I'm disclaiming speaking for the health insurance industry or even The Travelers, for that matter. The CBO people have discussed the various options that are in front of you, and there are a lot of experts in this room in the health delivery and financing area who have read or attended the congressional hearings and probably read the entire green books.

A lot of the material that has been put out was developed on the basis that there is a crisis, but the developments of the last 18 months have changed all that, at least, I think, from a political standpoint.

From trust fund insolvency, perhaps by this year, according to estimates of a couple of years ago, we're looking for insolvencies not before the year 2000, which is hard for politicians or even regular people to deal with.

So the driving force at this point in policy changes is not going to be the trust fund insolvency threat. More of the discussion has to do with the impact of Medicare on the overall federal budget, the percentage of gross national product that health takes up, and the impact of health costs on the competitiveness of American employers' goods and services. Also, perhaps, in this environment the options will be addressed more on the basis of logic than on some kind of a quick fix.

How Health Insurers View the Options

Our industry, the health insurance industry, has kept a pretty open mind on the various options for dealing with Medicare financing issues. The things that make the most sense to us, or at least to me, include increasing the percentage of Part B, SMI outlays that are paid by beneficiaries versus the general revenue contributions.

We would also agree with the introduction of income-related cost sharing, and there are a lot of proposals around about this. This could be done either through the taxing system or through the premium. As Karen Williams mentioned, we wouldn't recommend income-related benefit determinations, a pretty messy situation.

We also looked at the question of means testing eligibility, and we would not be in favor of that. In the long run, we might be able to move to means testing, but this would have to be accompanied by some incentives for people to save for private health insurance and for some other guarantees that affordable private benefits would be available.

Sheila Burke referred to the shifts of costs to employers through the ESRD program and the working-aged provisions. This has been done without too much of a complaint from the employer community in this country, but I think there is a limit to how far shifting Medicare costs to employers can go. Certainly major incentives would have to be established for employers to maintain retired health plans primary to Medicare.

This would not be infeasible today. Obviously, employers would drop the retired health plans if that's what it took. So, if retired employee health plans are to be a long-term approach, there would have to be major incentives established.

I've been participating with a Business Roundtable staff group which has been studying Medicare reform issues for about the last year. Again, the climate has changed substantially during that period— from impending trust fund doom to relative calm.

In connection with that activity, I asked some actuaries at Travelers to look at the possibility of all the future cost increases under Medicare being absorbed by the beneficiaries, either through taxing the beneficiaries or by cost sharing premiums or benefits.

We made an assumption that the federal government would continue to add to its Medicare expenditures from the 1983 base on the basis of growth in the economy and the increasing number of Medicare beneficiaries. All other costs in that assumption would be shifted to the Medicare beneficiaries.

We reached the conclusion that you can't push all the future increases in Medicare over to the beneficiaries. For example, in 1983 dollars, using moderate assumptions to completely support the growth in Medicare expenditures beyond growth in the economy and the increasing number of beneficiaries, premiums would have to increase from the present $15.50 level to $74.29 by the year 2000. In current dollars, that's a 420-percent increase.

In nominal dollars, of course, the increase was much larger than that. That leads to the conclusion that Medicare financing must be addressed through a combination of increased beneficiary payments, reduced payments to providers either driven by competitive systems or otherwise, and, if necessary, increased taxes.

Concerning benefit changes: a lot of the thinking that I have seen combines increases in Part A and Part B cost sharing with the addition of a catastrophic benefit plan.

The idea, of course, of increased cost sharing is to induce more cost-effective health care, while the catastrophic feature will provide security for those who are really ill. It seems to me, at least, that these two subjects should be addressed separately. I think we should go forward with some increases in cost sharing, both to save money and to exert some downward pressure; but I'm not sure that adding a new benefit like catastrophic would be a good idea.

Depending upon the description of that catastrophic plan, once you reach the point where Medicare or any benefit plan is paying 100 percent of all of the charges, you have some incentives for the kind of heroic care here that we worried about earlier in this program.

This is a difficult problem with a regular employer group plan, and could be even more difficult with the Medicare group. So I wouldn't say that it couldn't be done, certainly; but I think there are cost considerations, and I haven't seen those fully examined.

The questions of technology and when and where new applications should be reimbursed under Medicare would be involved also, in that connection and as a freestanding question.

There aren't easy answers with respect to technology. I've heard arguments put forth well by the manufacturers of medical technology, and they make a very good point, that there are a lot of cost savings that go on right up to this moment that are driven by improved technology. On the other hand, some of the potential applications for technology in terms of expenditures are mind boggling, with respect to the breadth of the population they could reach.

I think we need a balance here that doesn't impede research and development, but provides for a rational decision-making process as to when and where technology should be applied. To a great extent, looking at Medicare financing is really looking at hospital expenses and where they are going.

For a number of years, the insurance industry has favored all-payer hospital prospective reimbursement programs established under state law. This policy grew out of the combination of tremendous hospital inflation and questions of equity with our friendly Blue Cross competitors. This policy has, I think, been a positive one for our industry, and has made a positive contribution to raising the total national awareness of health cost inflation.

I also think that the health insurance industry's work directly contributed to the enactment of the federal DRG program. But after a few years, now, we have the federal DRG program, and we have 10 states that have some form of all-payer systems.

Again, we have felt all-payer was important, because it precludes the possibility of costs being shifted from the control group to a noncontrol group of patients. But ironically, I think that our work on the hospital cost containment bill proposed by the Carter administration in 1979 and on the ultimate DRG bill has moved us to a point where further state developments in the all-payer area are becoming less and less likely. Certainly, obtaining Medicare waivers will be less and less likely.

So as we move very quickly away from cost and charge reimbursement to the DRG environment for Medicare and a multiple contracting environment for a growing number of the rest of the patients, policy questions do arise which affect Medicare and all other payers and patients.

One of the questions relates to uncompensated care. This has always been a major concern to insurers because of cost shifting, but, at least from a public interest viewpoint, as long as charge-based patients would bear the freight, care could be rendered.

Now with Medicare and the hospitals themselves squeezing reimbursement from Medicare patients, and more of the other patients moving away from charge-based reimbursement, the actual provision of care is being threatened, and charge-based paying patients and third-party payers are facing even greater cost shifting. We need more thinking into the alternatives, legislative and otherwise, which we can use to address the uncompensated care situation.

Alternative Financing Arrangements

Medicare is also at the heart of the new competitive arrangements by encouraging HMOs and other arrangements to serve as alternative financing and delivery arrangements for Medicare beneficiaries.

Alternative financing arrangements are directly related to the overall issue of Medicare financing and the future status of the trust funds. The question is: will the new HMO arrangements which are at the heart of the administration's long-term strategy for Medicare help or hurt the trust funds?

Our industry has been looking at the question of Medicare opt-outs or vouchers for many years. Each time we've looked at this issue, we've concluded that voluntary opt-out programs would hurt the trust funds rather than help them.

There are two reasons for this. The first is adverse selection. We believe it's clear that, if you pay the HMOs and other opt-out plans 95 percent of the average per capita outlay for Medicare, you're paying too much in relation to the average usage for those who elect the opt-outs.

We know that an awful lot of Medicare outlays are concentrated on a small number of people. I think 10 percent of the population uses about 65 percent of the total outlays with a lot of expenses going into the last year of life.

In general, we think the younger and healthier Medicare beneficiaries will elect the new offerings. Further, a complicated issue beyond the initial adverse selection is the possibility of the people who do opt out into the HMOs opting back in when they become older and less healthy.

In sum, our industry has concluded that a mandatory opt-out might save dollars, but that a voluntary program wouldn't. At least, that's our thinking at this point in time.

The other problem with the current program is the cost shift. With a 20-percent-plus claim payment disadvantage against charges, only those third parties that can bargain for substantial discounts would participate in the Medicare programs. This will restrict competition.

In this regard, there's a further policy question regarding who controls the HMOs and other third-party arrangements being offered to Medicare beneficiaries.

It has seemed clear to me, at least, for some time that the providers have a unique advantage when they also become the financers of care. So when national hospital chains announce that they're going into financing of medical care and will have millions of people under their plans within five years, it seems to me that they also recognize the unique advantage that a provider has when it gets into financing.

First, of course, there would be no need for a provider group to negotiate arrangements with providers for discounts or for more favorable utilization arrangements. For nonprovider organizations entering the HMO-PPO field, these negotiations are critical to their success or failure.

I would ask the question in general also, if we had a problem when providers controlled only delivery, will quality, cost, and access work out to the public good when providers control a large share of both financing and delivery?

Finally, in my paper I referred to excess hospital capacity. This excess is large now. It's growing, and we're going to go through quite a wrenching process here as—in dealing with the issues of hospital competition—we see which hospitals are going to be hurt in terms of the competitive arrangements.

To the extent that hospitals that are providing uncompensated care or providing needed teaching or other public interest functions get hurt, public policy choices must be made to deal with needed services.

Discussion

Income-Related Benefits and Premiums

MR. JACKSON: It seems to me that both speakers have rejected income-related benefits as being impractical. I just wonder why an income-related deductible, for example, at the front end is considered so impractical. If the deductible at the front end is not income related, it seems to me it's less fair. It falls more heavily on the person with low income than on the person with high income.

MR. TROY: I think, basically, it's not a philosophical matter. It's a matter of the administration of the plan. In other words, if you have income-related benefits, then you have the possibility of 28 million people with different benefit plans. It's a lot easier to administer through the premium process than through the taxing process. It's not a philosophical argument, really.

MR. KITTREDGE: John, you might contrast it with the employer-type plan which does have an income-related deductible, but one which is based upon what the employer's payment is to the employee. That's easy to determine. To try to determine the Medicare recipient's income, which really comes from a variety of sources, is, I think, a much more difficult thing to do.

MR. JACKSON: You can get his tax return from the last year.

MR. TROY: Of course, the other problem is the breadth of it. If you have an income-related premium, you're going to hit everybody. If you have an income-related benefit, you're only going to hit those in the category that have a claim. So the premium is a broader source of revenues, in any event.

MS. DEIGNAN: I was thinking about some of the issues of income-related contributions before and, since you brought it up now, let me say I would agree basically with what you said, that anybody in Congress who is trying to evaluate options for any kind of means testing or income-related contribution to Medicare first has to face the fact that there is no good proxy for income for the elderly that could be used.

Basically, if you wanted to do a very fair and an even income-related test within Medicare itself, you would have to go back to ground zero and begin requiring declarations of assets, income, et cetera, at the point of determining eligibility for the program or some other point.

Now, that is a concept that has absolutely no relationship with the Medicare program now. Those are the kinds of problems that lead to the general statements of administrative infeasibility or difficulty, in applying income-related concepts to Medicare. The amount of an individual's Social Security check, or the taxes he or she pays, are not necessarily good indications of total income or ability to contribute more to the cost of medical care.

There have been varying opinions on whether or not any kind of a means test could be done, or should be done. I personally tend to agree that it's going to be almost impossible whether or not one makes a judgment that that should be done. But I would also like to point out that when you begin to get serious discussion in Congress of some kind of means test, whether it's through the tax system or something else, it basically begins to surface in relationship to discussions about increases in beneficiary cost sharing.

You find that people who would normally not even consider anything like that begin to get worried on the other side when they see that the cost sharing is going up. They worry about whether some people are going to be able to bear that increased cost sharing that is already built into Medicare.

So it is natural to look for ways to try to protect those lower-income groups. I think you'll begin to see more and more members of Congress thinking about it in those terms. Whether or not that makes the issue of administrative feasibility any easier is another question. I don't see necessarily that it does. But I would also like to point out that there is a very small provision in the law now which shows that happening a little bit already. The premiums were increased in Medicare over the last couple of years, because of the fear of having monthly Social Security checks reduced since the premiums are deducted directly from Social Security checks, and a provision in the law now says, in effect, that people with low Social Security benefits will not have the same premium increase or pay the same premium that other high-benefit receivers do.

The reason for doing that was to prevent reduction in monthly Social Security checks, but one could also make the point that that is an income-related feature in the program already. It's very small. It wasn't done for that reason, but it's there.

Means-testing options are inextricably related to concern about increases in cost sharing.

64

The Impact of Medicare Reform on the Private Sector

Paper by Cynthia K. Hosay

Title XVIII of the Social Security Act—known as Health Insurance for the Aged and Disabled, but more commonly called Medicare—will mark 20 full years of operation in July 1986. The massive program, enacted on July 30, 1965, but not operational until July 1, 1966, was born in the midst of heated debate and has functioned in controversy ever since.

Part of that controversy has been generated by the giant scope of the program. In 1984, over 29 million people were covered by Medicare at a cost of approximately $65 billion. During 1985, some 31 million enrollees will receive benefits under the program at an anticipated cost of $70.8 billion. As the cost of medical care has risen, and the number of aged Americans eligible for Medicare has grown, the cost of the program has soared.

While current estimates suggest that the system will remain solvent until 1998—assuming moderately favorable conditions—and may even maintain itself into the next century if the economy is favorable, there is little disagreement that Medicare requires rethinking as it approaches its 20th year.

The latest report of the Advisory Commission on Social Security, which was submitted to the Secretary of Health and Human Services in March 1984, focused on an impending Medicare "crisis." Since then, a host of authorities, including Robert Ball and Robert Meyers, formerly of the Social Security Administration, Wilbur Cohen and Dr. Karen Davis, formerly of the Department of Health, Education and Welfare, and various congressional staff members, elected officials, private organizations, and academicians have directed considerable attention toward developing "solutions" for Medicare.

This paper focuses on four suggestions that have received considerable attention and appear to have important implications for the private sector. None of these considers building more accountability into the health care system as, say, the DRG system does. Rather they focus on:

- changes in employer plans;
- taxation of supplemental insurance;

65

- provision of supplemental catastrophic coverage by the government; and
- adoption of medical equivalents of the individual retirement account.

Each of these concepts is examined by asking three questions:

(1) What is being proposed?

(2) How would the private sector be affected by the proposal?

(3) How would Medicare beneficiaries be affected?

Employer Plans

The first set of proposals for reform focuses on employer-provided health benefits for older and retired workers and their spouses. Studies show that most large companies and many smaller ones provide medical coverage for such workers since Medicare coverage is modest. The federal program covers only about 45 percent of total health care outlays of the elderly, according to Dr. Karen Davis. The nature of that coverage varies. Most companies pay for expenses not covered by Medicare, but do not pay for services outside Medicare's scope. Thus, employer outlays for these plans, though significant for employers, may also be modest relative to total health costs of retiree families.

Consequently, almost any proposal to alter Medicare financing or benefits will affect most employers at least indirectly.

In addition, several administration proposals extend employers' health insurance coverage both to elderly spouses of nonelderly workers and to elderly workers themselves. Those proposals would accelerate a trend to make employer-provided health insurance coverage primary. In 1982, the Tax Equity and Fiscal Responsibility Act (TEFRA) required that health insurance offered in the work place serve as first (or primary) payer for workers aged 65–69 covered by the plan. Medicare, formerly the primary carrier, became secondary.

In 1984, the Deficit Reduction Act (DEFRA) required employers to offer the coverage to spouses, aged 65 through 69, of employees under age 65. The coverage, if elected, is primary to Medicare.

As part of its fiscal year 1986 budget proposal, the administration proposed that employees over age 69 be allowed to choose the employer-sponsored plan as their primary coverage, making Medicare secondary (this proposal would extend current law applying to workers age 65 to 69).

A second factor to consider is the proposals made by the administration, the Congressional Budget Office, the Advisory Council on

66

Social Security, and others to increase the amount beneficiaries pay in premiums, copayments, or deductibles. Since many employer plans pay for the Medicare Part B premium as well as the deductible and copayments required of beneficiaries, those employer-sponsored plans would be directly affected by such proposals to increase cost sharing.

At the same time, costs to employer plans could well increase simply because more workers are living longer after they retire. Thus, employers who supplement Medicare would pay a larger share of the cost of care for a growing number of people.

A third proposal that would have had direct implications for employers is the proposal to tax health insurance premiums that exceed $70 a month for an individual and $175 for a family. That proposal, made by the Advisory Council on Social Security and endorsed by Robert Ball, former commissioner of Social Security, could earmark a portion of the tax revenue for the health insurance trust fund. To the extent that some employer plans continue the same coverage that a retired worker had when he or she was working, those premiums might be subject to the tax.

While the new Reagan proposal to tax the first $10/month for individual and $25/month for family premiums paid by the employer seems to have little impact on employer-sponsored plans, several questions remain. First, would employer-paid Medigap premiums also be taxed? Secondly, if the employer pays the premium for Medicare Part B, would that be taxed?

Just when employers are being asked to accept greater liability for the health care of older and retired workers, some courts have interpreted the employer's promise of health benefits as a sacred pledge (White Farm decision; Bethlehem Steel). A move to create a vested right to health benefits would do nothing to ease the employers' burden.

There are two more possible, contradictory developments that should be mentioned in a discussion of how proposals to reform Medicare would offset employer plans. One is a proposal by the Financial Accounting Standards Board that employers report a liability for the future costs of retiree health benefits that are not offset by assets to pay for them. The second is a limitation on tax-exempt contributions to reserves under the Deficit Reduction Act—a step that discourages prefunding.

In sum, certain employers may conclude that their only option is to cut back on their coverage of older workers and retirees by cutting benefits for all.

Should Congress pursue this route to its farthest limit and make employer plans primary in all cases, costs in the private sector would certainly rise. If future court decisions eliminate the possibility of modifying benefits for retired workers, such benefits would inevitably require prefunding. Restricting tax deductions for the prefunding of benefits would put heavy pressures on companies providing coverage for elderly employees or retirees.

If, however, the employer plans could remain as secondary payer for retired workers, benefits provided under the employer's plan would be viewed as supplemental, or Medigap, insurance.

Medigap Insurance

The Congressional Budget Office estimates that nearly two-thirds of the elderly and disabled are currently covered by some form of private insurance to supplement Medicare. In addition, approximately 14 percent are covered by Medicaid.

It is not clear exactly how many employer plans supplement Medicare or pay for the cost of Medigap insurance but several recent studies indicate that between 60 and 85 percent of employer-sponsored plans continue some form of coverage after normal retirement age to supplement Medicare. Coverage is rare, however, in small group plans (less than 100 employees). It is estimated that approximately one-quarter of employer-sponsored plans providing coverage to retirees pay for the Part B premium. Others offer a Medicare carve-out and still others a Medicare supplemental policy.

Medigap coverage varies, but generally pays all or part of the deductible and coinsurance for hospital insurance, and may pay the 20 percent copay portion of Part B supplementary medical insurance, covering physicians' charges.

Perhaps the best-known Medigap insurance is that offered by the American Association of Retired Persons. It covers some hospital, medical, surgical, and skilled nursing facility services that are partially covered by Medicare. Like most Medigap policies, many forms of service that are frequently required by older people are not covered. Excluded are outpatient dental care or dentures, check-ups, routine footcare, immunizations, eye examinations, and the cost of eyeglasses and hearing aids. Since Medigap policies supplement Medicare, and Medicare does not cover intermediate or custodial care in a nursing home, neither do most Medigap policies.

The Congressional Budget Office noted three reasons that Medigap insurance is sought. The first is that coinsurance amounts may accumulate for those who use Medicare-covered services extensively.

Secondly, there are gaps in Medicare coverage—particularly for nursing home care. Finally, Medicare offers little protection against catastrophic illness.

Yet, the Congressional Budget Office, Robert Ball, and others have proposed a tax of 30 percent on premiums for Medigap policies that pay any part of the first $1,000 of Medicare's required cost sharing. They argue that holders of supplemental coverage are shielded from the cost of care and use more health services. They also maintain that "since Medicare actually pays for much of increased medical care use that results from private insurance coverage, the price of private insurance does not fully reflect the costs of higher use" (CBO, Feb. 1985). Medicare, then, is liable for 80 percent of the increase.

Taxing premiums would raise the cost of Medigap coverage and discourage the purchase of such coverage so as to retain incentives for beneficiaries to attain lower utilization.

Clearly, those who would suffer most would be lower-income beneficiaries. The millions who have no supplemental coverage are likely to grow in number since the increase in premiums for Medigap policies could well deter the purchase of such coverage by many who now have it.

Those employer plans that pay Medigap premiums for their retirees would also be negatively affected by imposing a tax on Medigap premiums. Other employer plans, which supplement Medicare coverage by extending plan coverage to older and retired workers, could also be regarded as Medigap insurance and become subject to taxation.

As Senator Lloyd Bentsen remarked in introducing a bill to create a federal Medicare supplemental insurance plan, ". . . about 10 million elderly persons have no Medigap insurance and face catastrophic risks because, for many, the average monthly premium of between $40 and $50 is insurmountably high."

Federal Government Supplementation of Medicare

A third proposal for Medicare reform addresses the lack of protection against catastrophic illness under Medicare. Currently, the Medicare program is designed to finance acute medical care, but the diseases of old age are often chronic in nature. With its emphasis on acute care, Medicare provides weak protection against catastrophic expenses resulting from lengthy illnesses or costly treatment modes.

Several proposals have been made to place a "cap" on patient liability for covered Medicare expenditures. That cap would protect patients from costly hospital stays or large physician bills that can wipe out savings.

One such proposal (CBO report *Reducing the Deficit*) would increase cost sharing for Medicare Parts A and B, and add a Medicare Part C to provide for catastrophic protection. Medicare Part A pays toward hospital, skilled nursing, and home health care services. Part B pays toward physicians' services and hospital outpatient services. Both have their own financing, deductibles, and copay provisions.

The cost-sharing provisions of Medicare Parts A and B would be coordinated so that out-of-pocket liability under either part would be limited to $2,000. Part C, the catastrophic benefit, would be financed by a separate premium. All Medicare participants who elected Part B would be required to elect Part C as well.

If such a program were implemented on January 1, 1986, the premium for Part B would be $200 and for Part C $75, according to Congressional Budget Office estimates.

The deductible amount under Part B would increase. Copayments for most enrollees not using hospital services would also increase under this proposal. Preliminary estimates show that less than 1 percent of enrollees who did not use hospital services would benefit from the cap on copayments. Twenty-three percent of enrollees using hospital services and 5 percent of all enrollees would benefit from the catastrophic cap in 1986.

But enrollees would still be liable for disallowed charges, noncovered services, and premium costs for both Part B and Part C. Since the private sector frequently pays for part or all of uncovered costs (premium, copayments, deductibles, and uncovered charges), the private-sector costs could be expected to increase.

Yet another idea was advanced by Senator Bentsen. He proposes that the federal government provide optional coverage for the 20-percent coinsurance requirement of Medicare Part B. That coverage would be financed by an additional premium. Senator Bentsen's proposal would increase costs to the plan for employers who pay only the premium costs. But for plans that pay the 20-percent coinsurance, such a program might actually reduce costs significantly.

"Medical Individual Retirement Accounts"

Finally, some have proposed that the responsibility for providing for the medical needs of the elderly be shifted away from government and returned to the individual. A proposal to establish and encourage universal individual health credit accounts (or "medical IRAs," as they have been called) has received attention from both the Heritage Foundation and the Advisory Council on Social Security.[1]

Stressing individual planning for private health insurance coverage in retirement, the Medicare system, under this proposal, would be restructured over a 30-year period to enable and require individuals to make provisions to pay for the bulk of their own medical bills, other than for catastrophic expenditures.

Current employer and employee Medicare taxes would be frozen and the government would establish a universal health credit account for all workers and their spouses. Those accounts would be available for workers and spouses to purchase basic care in their retirement. Some suggest that those accounts eventually would cover expenditures only over a fixed percentage of income.

In addition, workers would be encouraged to establish their own health IRAs through a tax credit or deduction for contributions to the IRA. The current Medicare tax paid by employers and employees would be used to provide Medicare benefits to current beneficiaries and, over time, to fund the universal health credit accounts.

Each worker would receive an annual statement of the value of his or her health credit account. After age 59½, workers and retirees could draw on the balance of their accounts to purchase medical insurance or actual medical care. Withdrawals from medical IRAs would be permitted for the same reasons.

Employees would be permitted to contribute up to $500 a year to their medical IRAs sponsored by employers, reducing employees' taxable income by the amount contributed. These employer-sponsored savings programs would be critical to the success of the medical IRA program since employers would be encouraged to match employee contributions.

Under the medical IRA proposal, the next 30 years would see another savings plan listed on the company benefit roster and add a new administrative burden. In addition, employers would continue to pay the Medicare tax to supply catastrophic coverage while perhaps contributing the maximum of $500 to the employees' medical IRAs.

Since the program is designed to encourage the purchase of individual health insurance policies, or direct payment for care, the ben-

---

[1] Editor's note: A brief discussion of universal individual health credit accounts can be found in Appendix B ("Executive Summary of Recommendations," *Medicare Benefits and Financing: Report of the 1982 Advisory Council on Social Security* (Washington, DC: U.S. Government Printing Office, 1983).) See Chapter VII, Section A, of the full report for a complete discussion.

efits of insurance may be diluted for all. (Insurance is predicated on shared risk.) Employers who choose to continue to provide health benefits for retired workers might then face higher premiums because of adverse selection.

Conclusions

In conclusion, one might reasonably ask whether the four proposals discussed have anything in common. If so, what?

First, it seems safe to say they would all have some impact on the private sector. I believe they all represent a shift from collective to individual responsibility that would impose higher costs on both employers and employees. Yet none of the proposals seek to control health care costs by altering the current system of delivering care. Cost sharing focuses on the demand side of the medical care equation. Physicians, hospitals, and other health care providers would be affected only indirectly by the cost-sharing requirements of their patients.

The Medicare crisis offers opportunities to reform Medicare in a fashion that would benefit government, beneficiaries, and employers by continuing to focus on provider practices and reimbursement. If the actual costs of providing care are contained by controlling the number and kinds of health services delivered and the costs of those services, all payers win.

Yet, the implications for the private sector of the four proposals to shift costs are important. They suggest that the private sector's burden would increase substantially while little would be done to control the costs of medical care for all payers.

Remarks of Cynthia K. Hosay

MS. HOSAY: I would like to say that my task today is not only a pleasure, it is really quite a challenge as well. There are two principal reasons why I say that. First, the very title of the presentation, "The Impact of Medicare Reform on Private Supplementation of Medicare," raises some intriguing questions.

One of them, of course, is that the word "reform," at least to me, always has a very positive connotation. If we are talking about some of the proposed reforms in terms of the private sector, however, and by the private sector I'm going to narrow it primarily to the employer sector, I would ask you to consider whether, in fact, "reform" is the correct term.

72

Then there are so many Medicare reforms that have been proposed that it is like standing on quicksand. Anyone who had a chance to glance at my first paper will notice that it's considerably outdated now, because it contains a long discussion about the tax cap. And some of the other reforms may fall into the same position.

The other reason why I find the topic a challenging one is that the private sector is by no means a monolithic organization or institution, as every one of you in this room knows. So, any reform that we consider today will have varying impacts, depending on the nature of the particular plan in question.

That being said, I'd like to focus on four particular reforms that have received considerable attention because they would, in fact, have a widespread and significant impact on the private sector.

Those four are, in very broad terms, changes in the nature of employer plans or coverage, the taxation of supplemental insurance, the provision for supplemental catastrophic insurance to be provided by the government, and, finally, the adoption of the medical equivalent of the individual retirement plan.

Changes in Employer Plans

The first set of proposals for reform focuses on employer-provided health benefits for both older and retired workers and for their spouses.

Some of us believe that there has been a trend toward the shifting of responsibility for health care coverage of those particular groups to the private sector. And, certainly, if you look at some of the recent changes in TEFRA that have been discussed, including the 1984 changes, you see that more and more the private sector is assuming responsibility—perhaps not willingly—for older workers, retired workers, and Medicare-eligible spouses of those two groups.

A proposal has been set forth by the administration to allow those over age 69 to be covered by the employer if that person is still working. That proposal would continue the shift toward employer responsibility.

Now, I recognize that there is a difference in interpretation between those of us who work with the private sector and the people in Washington who are "government related"—or perhaps it is a difference of perception—as to whether or not this shifting responsibility is a growing trend.

This trend is being forced to continue as the private sector is being asked to shoulder an increasing burden for older people. Employer plans are also covering more costs for older people simply because, as a result of an improved health care system, more and more people are living longer—which, we should note, is a wonderful comment on our society and our capabilities. In the midst of all of this doom-saying we ought not to forget that.

I have been planning to discuss the proposal to tax benefits over $70 and $175 a month. Instead, it is necessary to mention the newest proposal, which is to tax the first $10 a month for individuals and $25 per month for families.

The impact of that particular proposal on the private sector and employer plans may be far less initially than the tax cap would have been. Nevertheless, it is something that employers will want to watch very carefully to see how it evolves.

At the same time, Karen Williams talked about the notion that, just as employers are being asked to accept a greater liability for older people, some courts are interpreting the employers' promise of health benefits as a sacred pledge.

There are also two possibly contradictory developments of significance for the employer community. The first is the Financial Accounting Standards Board's [FASB] proposal that employers report a liability for the future cost of retiree health benefits that are not offset by assets to pay for them. FASB's proposal suggests a trend toward prefunding. The second, as we heard this morning, concerns the limitations imposed by DEFRA on the ability of employer plans to prefund adequately.

So it is something of a "catch-22." In fact, one might conclude that certain employers may find that their only option is to cut back on overall health benefit coverage in order not to risk charges of discriminating against groups of older employees.

These developments are certainly something to think about. If Congress pursues this route of encouraging employer liability at the limit, employer plans would be primary in all cases and costs in the private sector would certainly rise. If future court decisions eliminate the possibility of modifying benefits for retired workers, such benefits would inevitably require funding.

However, if the employer plan could remain as secondary payer for retired workers, benefits provided under the employer's plan would be viewed as supplemental, or Medigap, insurance.

Taxing Medicare Supplement Insurance

That raises the second issue to be considered today. That is: most of you know that an estimated two-thirds of people who are covered under Medicare, the elderly and disabled, have some kind of private supplementation. In addition, while roughly 14 percent are also covered under the Medicaid program, the rest does, in fact, come directly from the private sector.

Several people today have talked about the difficulty of determining the extent of private supplementation of Medicare. Studies I have seen, including a number conducted by groups represented in the room this morning, indicate that anywhere from 60 to 80 percent of employer plans supplement Medicare coverage in some way. What we do not know is how many provide supplementary coverage or the nature of that coverage. Depending on the study and the group surveyed, there are different estimates. And, depending on the questions asked by the survey, the information derived on the nature of supplemental coverage varies.

We do know, however, that most Medigap policies cover most or all of the deductible and coinsurance for hospital insurance. They may pay the 20-percent copay for Part B supplemental medical insurance, as well. The best-known Medigap policy is the one provided by the American Association of Retired Persons. Like many policies, it fills in gaps in what Medicare already covers. Services that are not covered by Medicare in the first place usually are not covered by Medigap policies, either. The one notable exception may be prescription drug coverage. Other than drugs, to the extent that Medicare does not provide adequate long-term care, home care, outpatient, dental, vision, and a whole myriad of other benefits, most Medigap policies do not cover those services either.

The proposal to tax Medigap insurance requires an understanding of why beneficiaries purchase supplementary coverage in the first place. Earlier, Steve Long mentioned three reasons.

First, it seems that coinsurance amounts tend to accumulate for people who use a lot of Medicare-covered services. Second, the gaps in Medicare coverage, particularly for nursing home coverage, encourage people to purchase additional coverage. Finally, we do know that Medicare covers very little in the way of catastrophic illness. Those are three very strong incentives for older people considering the likelihood of being sick and needing coverage.

Yet this proposal would impose a tax of 30 percent on premiums for Medigap policies that pay any part of the first $1,000 of Medicare cost sharing. Proponents of that tax argue that the holders of supplemental coverage are shielded from the cost of care and, therefore, they use more health services.

As we heard this morning, there are questions about who uses more services and whether or not they do have any discretion over the amount of services utilized. In spite of such questions, one of the underlying justifications given for the proposal to tax policies paying the first $1,000 of cost sharing is to attempt to alter utilization of services.

It is also maintained that, since Medicare actually pays for much of the increased medical care use that private insurance encourages, the price of private insurance does not fully reflect the increase in cost. Therefore, Medicare is thought to be liable for 80 percent of the increase in utilization and the private insurance sector only gets 20 percent of that liability. Consequently, taxing Medigap coverage would encourage people not to purchase Medigap coverage, and that might, in turn, the argument goes, encourage people not to use so many discretionary health services. Clearly, those who would suffer most would be low-income beneficiaries and those employer plans that pay Medigap premiums for their retirees.

Supplemental Catastrophic Insurance

A third proposal that has been discussed in some detail today would combine Parts A and B and add a Medicare Part C to cover catastrophic illness. All participants who elected Part B would be required to elect Part C.

Any plans that pay for Medicare premiums, and a number of plans seem to do so, would feel the impact of the increase in premiums. Their costs would inevitably rise.

"Medical IRAs"

The fourth and last proposal I would like to touch upon is the creation of "medical individual retirement accounts." In some ways, individual retirement accounts for medical expenses are the logical extension of the move toward shifting responsibility from government to the individual, if you will.

The proposal would establish universal individual health credit accounts for each Medicare beneficiary, and freeze the Medicare tax for both employees and employers so that, over the next 30 years, Medicare would become a catastrophic program covering only amounts over a certain percentage of income level or perhaps over a fixed amount.

At the same time, employers would be encouraged to set up individual medical savings accounts for employees who could then plan ahead for retirement. Employees could deposit $500 a year tax sheltered or tax credited into that account. Employers would be encouraged to match the contribution. That proposal would clearly increase employers' costs.

These four proposals have two things in common. First, while we have not looked at them in detail, it is clear they would all have some impact on employer plans that currently supplement Medicare. In addition, plans that do not currently do so might be forced to provide coverage whether they wanted to or not. The second common factor that I want to stress in my last remaining seconds is that none of these proposals seeks to control health care costs by altering the current system of health care delivery. Cost sharing focuses on the demand side of the medical equation. Physicians, hospitals, and other health care providers would be affected only indirectly by the cost-sharing requirements of the patients.

As Medicare turns 20, I believe there is a marvelous opportunity to re-examine the premises on which it was established. That opportunity could provide true reform, not only for the Medicare program, but also for some of the problems employers are facing in trying to manage health care costs. By encouraging care that is appropriately provided, by limiting services to those that are necessary and appropriate, and by assuring that the costs for those services are controlled, Medicare reform could have a positive impact on both the private and public sectors.

The implications for the private sector of the four proposals to shift costs are indeed important. They suggest that the private sector's burden would increase substantially, while little is being done to help the private sector to control the costs of medical care.

Medicare Reform: Where the Emphasis Should Be

Paper by John C. Rother

In 1985, 20 years after the enactment of Medicare, our health care system is in a period of rapid change. Medicare must also continue to change and so anticipate and guide the direction of more systemic changes. Without reform, older Americans face a continued weakening of their insurance protection and insufficient benefit coverage in terms of their actual health care needs. Without change, our technological advances in health care may not benefit our aging population as fully as possible. To guard against this scenario, AARP proposes a seven-point health care reform plan designed to strengthen, simplify, and preserve solvency for Medicare, as well as to contain rising health care costs for all Americans.

Twenty years after its inception and despite staggering investments, Medicare is becoming a much weaker health insurance program. The reasons go beyond any budget-motivated efforts to transfer more costs onto the patient. At least seven factors account for this alarming situation:

- *Out-of-pocket costs to those covered by Medicare are increasing rapidly.* On average, persons over 65 pay $1,660 per year out-of-pocket for health care today, fully 15 percent of the mean annual income for that group. In fact, we are back where we started in 1965—the health cost crisis that led to Medicare's enactment was that costs equalled 15 percent of income for those over 65; as a consequence, many older persons were not receiving adequate health care. Now, even without additional increases in coinsurance, deductibles, and premiums, out-of-pocket costs are projected to rise to about 20 percent of income by the year 2000, and we face the same access issue as before Medicare.

  Remember, too, that these figures are averages, and thus mask the truly harsh impact that out-of-pocket costs have on the poor or near-poor or on those 20 percent of beneficiaries who are heavy users of health care services each year. These latter individuals incur higher than average out-of-pocket expenses because they tend to be liable for greater coinsurance and deductible costs.

- *The DRG reimbursement to hospitals under Medicare has unquestionably altered the behavior of physicians and hospital administrators—most noticeably reflected in an accelerated reduction in average length of stay.* Since the implementation of DRGs, the average length of stay for Medicare patients has dropped by almost two full days. While this important objective may be an encouraging sign, representing more efficient use of hospital resources, it can also mean that we are risking adequate care for the patient, particularly the elderly patient. If no attention is given to strengthening the postacute care structure for those who cannot care for themselves after a hospitalization, early discharge in the name of cost containment may result in even more costly readmission for the system and the patient and longer stays for the second episode.

Originally, Medicare was primarily designed as a hospital insurance program, but to continue this limited focus will narrow Medicare's protections and leave elderly patients facing a postacute "no-care zone." Continued emphasis on shortening hospital lengths of stay without the counterbalance of strengthened coverage for postacute care—particularly community-based and family-oriented care—is dangerously short-sighted. It is reminiscent of the fundamental mistake made 20 years ago in mental health policy, when mental patients were deinstitutionalized, in the name of more cost-effective and humane care, to an inadequately implemented alternative system—or nonsystem—of community care.

- *Concern over hospital costs generally and the DRG reimbursement system, which applies only to inpatient costs, has redirected medical procedures that were traditionally done on an inpatient basis to outpatient settings.* While this may or may not be more efficient for the health system as a whole, it has the effect of shifting costs from Medicare Part A to Part B, which offers much less comprehensive insurance protection for the beneficiary. Not only are beneficiaries liable for a 20-percent copayment under Part B, but physicians can and often do bill the patient directly for the balance of their fee over and above what Medicare considers reasonable. That practice is not permitted for the hospital under Part A. Seventy percent of Medicare beneficiaries who receive Part B reimbursement today are subject to these excess physician charges. Total beneficiary liability for physician services under Medicare now equals 60 percent of physician charges, an alarming figure that explains the significance of physician assignment and other Part B reforms to the beneficiary.

- *Due in part to advances in acute-care treatment, and in part to better health practices on the part of older persons, the pattern of illness among older persons is shifting from the acute to the chronic.* This is already true for older women, and men are now catching up. Consequently the needs of an aging Medicare population are also shifting to long-term care for those with chronic illness or disability. But, because Medicare was designed to be an acute-care program, it covers very little in the way of long-term health care. The program ends up paying for care provided in the often more expensive but less appropriate hospital setting than for a long-term care alternative. Since those with chronic illness are the greatest users of the acute care system as it is currently structured and paid for, we bear a heavy price both individually and systemically for Medicare's failure to insure, and thus permit better management of, the care for these persons.

- *Medicare has never covered some of the most expensive and widespread health costs associated with aging—prescription drugs, eyeglasses, dental care, and hearing aids.* For many people, aging is a process of growing dependency on these "spare parts." Costs associated with these needs usually cannot be efficiently insured through individual private insurance plans, so they are borne directly out-of-pocket. We estimate that aged Medicare beneficiaries must spend roughly $400 per year on average for these items, a particular concern for those low-income elderly who do not qualify for Medicaid.

- *Although we support cost containment efforts in Medicare, we are increasingly concerned about the lack of an equal program commitment to quality assessment.* It is a simple matter to cut costs if we don't care about the consequences; but if we are to achieve real improvement in our health care system, we must discover which procedures, in which settings, for which types of patients, produce positive results. This concern goes well beyond needed and structured technology assessment. We must ferret out the causes for variations in medical practice and treatment, and we need to assess the impact of various procedures upon the frail elderly as a unique and highly vulnerable population.

- *Despite the increasing array of health care choices available to the public and the industry's embrace of competition rhetoric for health reform, consumers still lack essential price and quality information that would enable them to make informed choices.* Without provider-specific price and quality data, consumers will be powerless to "reward" the best providers or "punish" the worst. Market-based strategies for Medicare and system-wide reform are not credible without the necessary base of consumer information. The present program does not provide that data. Newly issued regulations under the peer review organizations (PROs) which provide for hospital-specific data have the potential for helping to close this gap and their implementation bears monitoring.

AARP's membership is deeply concerned about each of these factors which contribute to Medicare's weakness. In our internal surveys of the concerns of our members, we find that they want meaningful and comprehensive insurance coverage for health expenses and that they are willing to pay premium dollars to get it. Health expenses are the major unpredictable expenses facing retired persons on fixed incomes, and they want those expenses in a predictable, budgetable form—namely premiums—rather than in direct cost-sharing forms tied to their state of health, which they cannot predict. Moderate- and low-income older persons are most concerned about direct out-of-pocket liability for uncovered items such as drugs, eyeglasses, and hearing aids, while middle-class older persons are more likely to be concerned about the lack of Medicare coverage for long-term care expenses, which are increasingly understood to be the true catastrophic risk faced by the elderly. Confusion about the current Medicare benefit structure is fairly widespread, especially on the issue of extra billing by physicians and the lack of coverage for long-term care services. Finally, older people share a fundamental concern that they, through Medicare, remain an integral part of mainstream health care in this country, and not become a disadvantaged part of a tiered system with its separate reimbursement levels or levels of care.

In response to these needs for change in the health care system and to the concerns of our membership, AARP proposes a seven-point plan for Medicare reform. This plan is not incorporated as yet into any single legislative proposal, but it undergirds the range of our considerable activities in health policy at both the federal and state levels. In brief:

(1) *Medicare must be recognized as part of an overall health care system.* Reimbursement reform applicable to Medicare should extend to all forms of payment for care given to Americans of all ages. We need to prevent a tiered system and assure an equal playing field for all. For that reason, we not only favor state-based all-payer systems of hospital cost containment, but are also willing to see Medicare assume its share of responsibility for the costs of providing care for those who cannot pay and have no insurance as part of that all-payer system.

(2) *Reimbursement reform is the key to Medicare's role in cost containment.* However, while Medicare reimbursement should be neutral with regard to the setting in which care is delivered—in other words, it should not continue to favor institutional care—it must also pay a fair price for services given. Medicare reimbursement to physicians—the true decision makers on health care utilization—should be raised in many primary care situations, for example, to more fairly compensate for the care received. But with reasonable reimbursements, doctors electing to treat Medicare patients should then agree to accept assignment— that is, accept Medicare's "reasonable charge" as payment in full. Price setting for hospitals may need to be combined with volume measures in reimbursement formulas to prevent "gaming" of DRGs.

(3) *Current gaps in coverage must be addressed, generally by reallocating existing resources.* Savings from shortened hospital stays should be reinvested in postacute care, drug coverage, and prevention programs. Medicare coverage should include both nursing home care and in-home and community-based health services for those who can remain independent of institutional care. Medicare benefits should also include respite care to aid family caregivers and enable them to continue their efforts. Unless Medicare is changed into a truly comprehensive health program, it will not be able to manage the increasingly dynamic interactions between acute- and chronic-care needs, between formal and informal caregivers, and between care for illness and attention to wellness and health promotion.

(4) *Since health care costs will inevitably continue to outpace gains in payroll tax revenues, additional income will be necessary for Medicare.* We favor dedication of a substantial part of tobacco excise taxes to Medicare for

the reason that smoking is clearly associated with increased health problems. Thus, raising the tax on smoking is roughly equivalent to instituting a risk-related premium. We do not favor any additional increases in payroll taxes, since such escalation will only further stymy the creation of new jobs, which are essential to the economy.

(5) *Quality assessment research and measurement programs must be built into Medicare.* At present, we do not know enough about how to use Medicare to encourage or preserve quality health care, and cost-containment efforts that are insensitive to quality concerns put patients at risk. We support the use of a small percentage of Medicare funds for research focused on quality assessment. To advance the state of knowledge on the issue, AARP is sponsoring a conference later this year with the American Medical Association, the American Hospital Association, and the American Nurses Association on quality-of-care concerns.

(6) *Beneficiaries must have meaningful information if they are to play a constructive role in the evolution of our health care industry.* We favor the public release of provider-specific price and quality information about hospitals, nursing homes, physicians, and other providers. Mechanisms should be developed to place this information in the proper context to assure that it is appropriately understood and meaningful.

(7) *Strategies to strengthen Medicare should be based upon social-insurance principles.* Insurance is by far the preferable method for financing health care, as it is the only mechanism that can spread the risk adequately while preserving individual dignity for the beneficiary. Savings approaches for funding health care are subject to criticism, both because the ability to save is so unevenly distributed and because savings can never adequately protect against catastrophic expenses. Welfare approaches will inevitably mirror our experience with Medicaid, in which comprehensive benefits have been undermined by insufficient reimbursement levels, leading to both a second-class system of care and the tragedy of family impoverishment before assistance is available. Means-testing approaches to Medicare would do nothing to solve the problem of rapidly rising health care costs; they would merely shift more of the burden of those costs onto the elderly.

In closing, let me identify more explicitly the areas in health care reform that, in my judgment, need to be addressed both by Medicare and by employers and insurers in the private sector. Employers share with older persons a tremendous stake in the future adequacy of Medicare. As long as Medicare alone provides inadequate health insurance coverage, employees will demand supplemental coverage for their retirement that is comprehensive. Likewise, pressures will intensify in the future for coverage in areas such as long-term care, where Medicare is now completely lacking.

It seems obvious to me that, whether or not Medicare's role is strengthened or allowed to be further diluted in the future, there nonetheless remains a common agenda for progress in health.

First, we have to focus much more clearly on what it is that we're buying with all our health care dollars—what is quality care and how can we measure it?

Second, we need to support innovative ways to finance and deliver more comprehensive health services, ways that permit the substitution of appropriate lesser-cost services for higher-cost institutional ones. Here I'm thinking of such innovations as the social health maintenance organization which is now being demonstrated in four locations around the country.

Third, we need to develop insurance coverage for the critical "post-acute" care period.

Fourth, we need to develop and disseminate more useful information about the performance of individual health care providers to the public.

Fifth, we need to continue development of a prevention and health promotion program.

Sixth, we should work together to rationalize reimbursement methods for physician services, to ensure the proper incentives for both cost-effective and quality care.

Finally, it seems that we can no longer postpone the need to rationalize health care and insurance protection for those with chronic illness and disability.

I believe that health care can be managed much better than at present, and managed for both cost containment and optimum health outcomes. Only when this management reality can no longer be denied can we expect Congress and the American public to support comprehensive reforms in Medicare of a comparable nature. Until then Medicare reform will, of necessity, be incremental and reliant on a partnership between the public and private sectors. The interest of present and future generations of health care consumers requires no less.

Remarks of John C. Rother

MR. ROTHER: I think I can summarize the thrust of my paper quite succinctly. I won't review the first section, which outlines some of the dynamic changes that we see going on in health care that demand a response from the Medicare program. I would like to just take a second, though, to review the fundamental premises of Medicare reform where our members are concerned.

How the Elderly View Medicare

AARP now represents 19 million people, so we essentialy represent American public opinion over the age of 50. We have a very active program of survey research, and we've found, not surprisingly, that as we've grown the attitudes and values of our membership exactly parallel the attitudes and values of the American population over the age of 50. And I believe it's safe to say on health care that there isn't that much difference between the American public's attitudes over the age of 50 and those under the age of 50.

In fact, we've just completed a major survey with Yankelovich, Skelly and White on that exact question—on the differences of younger adults and older adults with regard to both retirement and health questions. The perhaps surprising conclusion of this study is that there is no measurable difference whatsoever according to age. There is a difference according to income and perhaps all the talk about savings approaches and tax incentives and individual responsibility is pretty well confined to the top income brackets and has absolutely no support below that, regardless of age. I think that's an interesting piece of information.

As far as our membership is concerned, there are basically two fundamental values that underly our approach to health care reform. The first value is that health care for older people ought to be mainstreamed. We should not have a different system of health care for older people than is in place for the majority of all Americans. Sure, we finance it differently; but in terms of the kind of care that people have come to expect throughout their lives, there's a very strong preference, an overwhelming preference, that that be continued in the retirement years. I think that underlies many of the concerns that we have about reforms that would uniquely squeeze down on Medicare and that might, in effect, lead to a second-class form of care or such a great differential between what Medicare provides, what Medicare pays, and what's available to the private sector, that there really is a different standard of medicine. AARP is concerned that, as we institute various freezes, we certainly are pushing in that direction today.

The other principal concern that underlies most of our positions in this area is that our members want a strong and adequate program of insurance coverage. They're willing to pay for it. They prefer to pay through premiums, because that's a way of reducing the risk, or at least managing the risk; but they want adequate coverage. Because Medicare is not an adequate program, most older people are willing to go out and purchase private supplemental insurance. They're not willing to subject themselves to any serious degree of unmanageable risk in the form of cost sharing that's related to the incidence of illness.

People will do, I think, sometimes very uneconomical things in order to make that expense a predictable, budgetable expense. I believe that any effort to institute even greater amounts of cost sharing in Medicare will inevitably simply drive most people who can afford it to trying to insure that risk through private supplemental forms of insurance.

Older people, for quite rational reasons, are extremely risk averse. They're extremely concerned right now with those areas for which they cannot purchase insurance. Long-term care, perhaps surprisingly, was the number-one concern of our members when asked, if they could change Medicare in any way, what would they want to see changed? In the last two years, there's been a very dramatic increase in this concern. Today, our members' number-one response is: we would like to see Medicare cover nursing home and long-term care expenses. In the past, the answer to this question was always coverage of catastrophic hospital expenses or reductions in copays.

I think that's a rational response, particularly for middle-class persons in retirement. They can insure themselves against everything else except the one thing that could really wipe them out, which is a long nursing home stay.

Now there are a couple of promising experiments. AARP is engaged in one with Prudential in trying to develop a product that's going to be marketable on a third-party basis to our membership that might cover long-term care, including home health. There's also the social HMO demonstration program, also a very interesting phenomenon called life care communities, all of which are principally attractive to the older population because they manage the risk. These programs allow people to budget for what otherwise is a very unpredictable financial and health risk, chronic illness.

So those two values, that health care for older people ought to be part of a mainstream health care system, and that there ought to be insurance approaches that are strong and adequate and that truly cover the risks that older people face, are the fundamental concerns of our membership.

Evaluating Health Care and Benefits

I would just add to that, in terms of our staff perspective, I think we're increasingly concerned that in recent years we've focused so heavily on cost containment that we've not looked equally carefully at the question, what are we buying for our money? In other words, we haven't closely examined questions of quality of care, of appropriate utilization and, for that matter, just simply information about health care providers and health care outcomes.

Later this year we will cosponsor a major conference with the AMA, American Hospital Association, and American Nurses Association, focused on quality assessment. We feel this conference is necessary because we really are operating in the dark to a much greater extent than is healthy, and I think that that applies just as much to Medicare and just as much to private insurers as it does to the individual health care consumer. We see the development and dissemination of information that goes both to price and quality to the consumer. More adequate information is absolutely crucial to continue progress in developing a more efficient health care system.

Coverage Over Cost

Finally, I'd just like to touch on financing by saying that the rhetoric in Washington is seriously out of sync with the real concerns of health care consumers. All of our survey data indicate that people are quite anxious to have adequate health insurance and are willing to pay for it. And, in fact, the support for the present system of payroll taxes for Social Security and Medicare quite outstrips any measurable indication of support for income taxation or any other form of taxation we've got.

That's not to say we support increasing payroll taxes. We don't. But I do think it's remarkable the extent to which the public seems to be willing to support more adequate financing as long as that's deemed necessary for adequate health-care protection, and is completely resistant, from anything we can see, to the idea of increased direct cost sharing on the health consumer.

So I think, in terms of our membership concerns and in terms of what we think is good policy, we'll be continuing the fight for an insurance-based financing system that is comprehensive, that's universal, and that's truly adequate to meet the health care needs that older people actually face.

Discussion

Means Testing

MR. TROY: Refresh my memory. Where do you stand on the income-related premium question?

MR. ROTHER: Well, I think that means testing is subject to a lot of misunderstanding. I don't see any significant level of agreement between liberals and conservatives on this issue, because conservatives very often propose means testing as, in effect, a barrier to treatment. You're not in the program until you meet an income test, such as in Medicaid, whereas liberals very often talk about more progressive forms of financing, such as through the tax system, to pay for the universal program.

It makes a big difference. We would have serious problems with anything that imposes a barrier to service. In other words, conditioning the copayment or deductible, or eligibility for a particular kind of service on income would, in our view, push the Medicare program to be more like what Medicaid is today.

I don't think that's been a successful experiment that we want to copy. On the other hand, if we're talking about progressive forms of financing for Medicare, our first suggestion would be to look at instituting a more risk-based premium by, in effect, dedicating excise taxes from the sale of tobacco into the whole range of our health care programs, because I think that's a fairer way to do it, and I think that the combination of income from that source and continued progress on cost containment would get us down the road quite a few years before we really had to look elsewhere for additional revenues.

I might say that we looked, when I was in the Senate, very carefully at the idea of an income-tax surcharge dedicated to Medicare. I think you would be quite surprised at how few older people have income of a sufficient nature to really generate any meaningful revenues. It's an attractive idea in theory, but when you actually look at where the income is and how much income would be generated from a system like that, it doesn't help as much as you might think.

Targeting of Benefits

MS. MOON: I want to pick up on a point that was raised earlier. That's the issue of indirect means testing, or, more correctly, targeting of benefits. It's the flip side of what was earlier discussed about means testing.

I don't want to sound too positive about a means-testing approach. On the other hand, one point that Karen Williams indirectly raised is the question of whether some of the proposals to change Medicare are implicitly a type of means testing although perhaps not in the preferred direction. If beneficiaries are affected differentially by a proposal, there may be arbitrary impacts on some, as compared to the intentional targeting that occurs with regard to means testing.

In particular, raising the age of eligibility from 65 to 67 would, as Karen Williams dramatically pointed out, affect two different groups of people. One would include those who have some coverage from employers and who retired because they had plenty of resources and decided on their own to do so. But the second group may well have had bouts of ill health or unemployment prior to retirement and opted to take Social Security benefits on a reduced level because they had no other choice.

It seems to me, in a sense, that such a change in Medicare represents an implicit kind of means testing, but one that hurts those who cannot afford to buy supplemental coverage. Before we simply discard the discussion of means testing and say we don't want to do that, I think we ought to be very careful to recognize that many proposals do not treat everyone equally and may be *worse* than means testing if they hurt individuals who can least afford to make other arrangements.

I would also like to raise the issue of cost sharing. Under Medicare, cost sharing for physician services is already very large, well above 20 percent. Such an amount is well in excess of what most people think is necessary to help control costs.

Coverage for Early Retirees

MR. KEENE: Karen Williams had some very interesting statistics pertaining to people who retired early and seemed to have no coverage. Then John Rother says that people are very concerned about predictable budgets, are risk averse and all that. I'm just wondering, how do we reconcile these two particular positions?

MS. WILLIAMS: I'd love to know what these folks are doing for protection. Maybe future data runs that Deborah Chollet and I try to work out will help to explain it.

We have some clues. We think something like 6 percent appear to be picked up by working spouses. As many as 15 percent might find themselves somehow eligible for military, VA [Veterans Administration], or CHAMPUS [Civilian Health and Medical Program of the Uniformed Services] benefits. Some others may be able to obtain group coverage through professional or religious affiliations and other associations.

I really don't know what's happening to these people. I suggest that some are now being continued by employers, maybe as many as 50 percent. But we think those continued are obtaining coverage through higher premium contributions and perhaps reduced benefits, although basically they receive the same plan as active employees. I suspect that a good share of early retirees are going self-insured— that is, taking the risk. We may see their costs picked up in the uncompensated care burden.

I think it really is shocking that we don't know what has happened to these folks. I also think there's a dynamic in progress that has a very good chance of eroding current levels of employer coverage. As John Troy pointed out, the shake-up that's happening right now in price competition and financing may erode the existing care net. It would be nice if we could get better data on these people before we move too far down the road in terms of these kind of changes.

Cost Shifting

MS. MYDER: I need to bring up means tests. It seems to me that, whether it's in this room or outside of the room, the question more important than means testing has not been fully answered. That is, do we want to increase cost-sharing levels? Is that the desirable way to go at this point?

When we're talking about means testing, whether it's the premium or the deductible or eligibility, we are talking about cost shifting. In the last couple of years, there's been quite an outcry, from privately insured groups and others in the private sector, that federal costs are being shifted, and indeed they have been and they still are. It seems to me that we're assuming that this will continue, and we're just trying to figure out ways to do it best.

I very strongly agree with one of Dr. Hosay's last comments, and that is, we're really not talking enough about changing the delivery or the financing of the health care system either to spend less or, as John Rother said, get our money's worth.

I think that we eventually will have to answer questions about means testing, but I think we need to look at some other things first.

We are discussing options, and certainly increasing cost sharing. Whether it's the beneficiaries' costs or whether it's the private sector's costs is an option; but I think we ought to be looking at some priorities, too. I don't hear enough discussion on how we will make physicians render services to people, old and young, more efficiently. How can we be sure that the money we spend is well spent? Later on, and only after reforms are instituted, if we discover we still need money, then we can look at some of these other options.

Income Levels of the Elderly

Ms. YOUNG: I'm wondering whether anyone has or is interested in undertaking some sort of verifiable study to give some idea of exactly where the income levels of the elderly are.

I see from Karen Williams' presentation and from the presentation here from the AARP that I'm beginning to, just from listening, suspect that what we have is almost no middle class, if I can use that term, because the middle class among the elderly has got to be at a much lower income level than middle class among the working people; there really may not be a very large middle section among Social Security recipients or retirees, but, rather, what we are seeing is a large number who have adequate resources and go and buy their condos in the Sun Belt and don't worry about where their health insurance is coming from. They buy it, if they retire early. And there is an equally large number of people who are very low-income and are having very great difficulties; just the coinsurance that they're paying for medical care, which is much higher than the 20 percent, is really just strapping them unbelievably. We really don't have any demographics to know who the senior citizens are and what income groups, because we average everything out. The average of somebody with a lot of income and a little bit of income turns out to be a medium range, but there may not be any people in that medium range.

Is anybody doing any statistical work at all?

MR. SALISBURY: I'm pleased to note, Leah, that EBRI has a study like that under way right now.

MR. SEIDMAN: In response to that point, I think that we tend to talk about the elderly as if they were a homogeneous group and so on. Of course, they are not.

The impact of the changes in Social Security, principally the changes since about 1970, has been to bring the percentage of the elderly in poverty to about the same as the rest of the population. But if you take those who are 25 percent above poverty, then you have a proportionately much larger percentage for the elderly than you do for the nonelderly.

In addition to that, you have to look at the age of the elderly. The older the population that you're talking about, particularly when you're talking about those over 75 and 80 and 85 and so on, first of all, the more likely they are single women—and the proportion of single women in general in poverty is much larger—and secondly, their income is related to a lower level of Social Security earnings. Even though the COLA [cost-of-living adjustment] has been applied to it over a period of time, it still means that they have a lower income.

I raise this to comment on the question of whether or not this is a risk-averse group and whether there's any contrast between the 62-to-65 group or the under-65 group and the fact that a large proportion of the over-65 group who are eligible for Medicare purchase the Medigap policies.

Unfortunately, we don't provide Medicare coverage at the time that people become eligible for Social Security. They have a three-year wait. Those people can't be risk averse. There's no way that they have of meeting their risk, at least until Karen Williams does her study, or whoever is going to do the study.

I think we've got to assume that. On the other hand, it's absolutely clear, and I think I certainly would agree with what John Rother has said, that to the extent that people can afford to do so—and I put "afford" in quotes, because they can't really afford to do so—they go out and buy these Medigap policies.

Now, the AARP and the National Council of Senior Citizens policies may be decent policies and really provide what these people need. There are an awful lot that are being sold that don't do them very much good.

Ms. WILLIAMS: The best document I've seen so far on the economic status of the elderly is in the Economic Report of the President that was released recently. From Leah Young's published article,[1] some of you know what I thought about the insurance section of that report, which is not much, frankly. But the first several pages of chapter 5 did the best job I've seen of compiling data from the Census, Medicare, and Social Security Administration, and from pension benefits on what is happening with the elderly and what are the trends. The propaganda doesn't start until about the last four pages. You have a really very useful document up to that point. Maybe someone will be able to come up with something better, but, in the short run, I think that's a good place to look.

---

[1] Editor's note: The reference is to "Reagan Criticized on Health Care Stance" by Leah Young (*Journal of Commerce*, 19 February 1985, sec. A, p. 1).

MR. ROTHER: As far as the income situation of the elderly goes, we've done about as much work there as on any other group in the population. And there's a wealth of data available, particularly from the Senate Special Committee on Aging. But in terms of what's important here, which is the health expenses of older people, there's a shocking lack of data.

It's very difficult, and I know because I've been trying, to correlate income with health expenditures. We do know that if you get a particularly long-term sickness you're in trouble very quickly on an income basis, and that health problems today, even under Medicare, are an economic threat just as much as a health threat. But we can't quantify it to nearly the extent that we can quantify income data.

The Politics of Medicare Reform Options

Remarks of Rep. Fortney H. (Pete) Stark

REP. STARK: I notice that my topic is the reform of the Medicare system, and I must admit in this group I come here with some trepidation. I'm new to the field of medicine, legislatively speaking. I really didn't pay much attention to it in my previous dozen years in the Congress and the Ways and Means Committee. The reason, I suspect, is that on the Public Assistance and Unemployment Compensation Subcommittee I was mightily involved in AFDC [Aid to Families with Dependent Children] and SSI [Supplemental Security Income] and Title XX,[1] where I've gathered some expertise, being tutored by Jim Corman.[2] That subcommittee is now being run ably by Harold Ford (D-TN).

It really never got quite so much attention. The Public Assistance Subcommittee doesn't have such a constituency as the Health Subcommittee. I've described that by saying that I've been the chairman now less than three months, and I have found that I have six organs that I was unaware existed. Each organ has a lobbyist. Most of them have a plastic replacement manufactured by somebody in Silicon Valley, and Humana has given me a card so that I can have it installed in me any weekend of my choice and charge it to my Visa card. So I am learning somewhat about the depth and breadth of the health care industry and the medical providers. I guess I'm going to be doing a bit of counterprogramming.

How Much Reform Is Necessary?

You're talking about how we should reform Medicare, and I would raise the issue as to really how much reform it needs at all. We in Congress tend to not react very quickly. We feel that it's better to do something later than sooner; if it ain't broke, don't fix it; if you stall long enough, it'll go away.

---

[1]Editor's note: Title XX of the Social Security Act provides for a federal program which reimburses states for the cost of providing social services to low-income persons.

[2]Editor's note: James C. Corman was a Democratic congressman from California and chairman of the House Committee on Ways and Means Subcommittee on Public Assistance and Unemployment Compensation.

I don't think that Medicare is broke in either sense of the word. There are complaints. Providers would like to be paid more and bothered less. The beneficiaries would like to pay less and be bothered less. But that's any government program, whether it's Social Security or the Post Office. By and large, I think there's a feeling that Medicare is doing a good job, a job that needs to be done, and doing it well.

We're in the middle of a revolution already. Before I got this new job, there was a rather drastic change made in the way we pay hospitals. I think we're going to make an equally drastic change in the way we pay physicians, but I don't think we've figured out how yet.

Between that and the budget process, which forces us into the posture of reacting, I don't think we've had any time to think about long-term reform or long-term improvement, or long-term payment for services that may become required in the future.

Equal Access to Health Care

One of my principal concerns and, I suspect, one of the concerns that Congress ought to face the soonest, is the people who don't receive medical care for whatever reason. Either they're too poor and they fall between the cracks of qualification or access, or, to a lesser extent all the time as we begin to build up a surplus of rooms and physicians, there's just not care available. I think that probably is being taken care of by the supply side of the economic equation.

The administration would like to turn this back not only to the states but get the government out of providing medical care. It's the theory of benign neglect. Or if you keep things in OMB [Office of Management and Budget] long enough, they will disintegrate. And you've seen that in a host of programs, and you've seen the results in rising unemployment and rising poverty and rising mortality among children of young, single mothers. It's very clear that, if you want to increase poverty and put the burden on the backs of the poor in this country, it's a very simple thing to do.

I think that this country and the system can provide care to everyone. The real problem is how it ought to be paid for. We are not the kind of people who can sit around and listen to horror stories of people dying on the steps of hospital doors that have been barred to them because they didn't have Gucci loafers on and they had no other identification to qualify them either as a participant in an insurance plan or as a well-to-do person.

HCFA and the Department of Health and Human Services attempt—and I'll get to that a little later—to stifle any progress in the legislative area by withholding information. I always think that's an interesting gambit for somebody in the legislative arena where we tilt with one another. I guess the theory is, if we don't have a report, we can't act. The fact is that we can legislate, and history will show that we often have acted with inadequate information. The results have sometimes been rather disastrous. So I think it's kind of a bad game of chicken to be playing both with your industry and the American people to say, "Well, we can't get the report out." The theory is that, therefore, we can't act.

Disproportionate-Share Hospitals

I'd like to turn to the topic of hospitals that serve a disproportionate share of poor patients, which is an area that I'm concerned about. It's quite obvious that David Stockman and his fellow piranhas in the budget office [OMB], who I often accuse of knowing the cost of everything and the value of nothing, have decided that making some adjustments for disproportionate care in institutions is not in the budget's best interest.

So they're not going to give us the information. We have had tremendously good cooperation from hospital associations in providing us with the information from the private sector. I think we're going to use it. I quite frankly see nothing wrong. Let's assume that we get a list of 600 hospitals that, on some basis, we can say would qualify as hospitals providing a disproportionate share of care to the poor and needy. Say somebody wants to swear under oath that those figures are straight. The danger is I might leave 30 hospitals out, because they don't belong to an association, or they don't want to divulge their figures. There are a lot of good reasons that they might not be in there, but it seems to me a whole lot better to err on the side of missing these 30 hospitals and giving the Secretary of HHS permission, if they meet the qualifications, to add them to the list later than to wait another couple of years to solve the problem—which, I would submit, on my subcommittee would probably come out with 11 of 11 votes.

I think there's a tremendous dissatisfaction on both sides of the aisle on our committee with the game that we're getting. I only wish I had Jake Pickle[3] here to explain the feeling in somewhat more graphic terms.

---

[3]Editor's note: J.J. Pickle (D-TX) is chairman of the Oversight Subcommittee, House Committee on Ways and Means; a member of the Health Subcommittee; and former chairman of the Social Security Subcommittee.

We are going to go ahead. I guess I would say to all of you and the people you represent that we will produce better legislation the more information we have. When we do the poorest job is when we really don't have good figures. There are a lot of cost figures, and almost no revenue figures. For us to really put both ends of the teeter totter into perspective, we need revenue figures. Then we have to know where the revenue comes from. Then we can begin to put together some fairly good decisions, which I think is better than acting in the blind.

So my prediction is that you're going to see in whatever package we bring forth, in response to our budget mandate, some assistance for disproportionate-share hospitals, and we're going to do it without Madam Heckler [HHS Secretary Margaret M. Heckler] and I think we'll probably do every bit as good a job. That may at least let us call off this nonsense of not having open communication between the executive and the legislative branches.

We used to believe that you had to use government health programs as a kind of wedge to change the whole system. I say that only after looking back over what my colleagues before me have suggested was a way to change the health care system.

I really don't see that. Take, for example, the issue of physicians' payments. I don't really see that as an issue that's going to be between the Congress and the AMA. I see that as an issue between the AMA and a group of hospitals and the Harvard MBA alumnae club. I really think that there will be some interesting dialogue between various professional and quasi-professional groups as to who's going to make the decisions in medical care delivery.

I think Congress is going to benefit. I think we're just going to sit back and watch the horses run to the barn and just hope we remember to duck our heads when we enter the door, because I don't necessarily think that the adversary relationship, as it's been traditionally assumed, is going to be between us.

It may very well, in my area, be between Kaiser[4] and other totally nonprofit operations and for-profit hospitals. Again, I would think perhaps the San Francisco Bay area residents would be the beneficiaries.

So I think, in this change that's come about with the large market and the large amount of money that's being spent in this country

---

[4]Editor's note: The reference is to Kaiser Permanente, an HMO health care provider headquartered in Los Angeles.

through Medicare, that the system itself will adjust and, I think, adjust quite well.

Medicare in the Future

When I said Medicare isn't broke in both senses of the word, we don't have any idea of what it will look like 10 years down the pike. I suppose some of it is easy to predict. We can plug in inflation numbers, and we can plug in the cost of real estate and the cost of bedpans, and, I suspect, the cost of medicine and the cost of a lot of things. But I don't think we can anticipate how much demand there is going to be as was generated by an article in *The New York Times Magazine* not so long ago, saying that we're doing a bum job because we're not providing long-term nursing home care.

Now that was really never part of Medicare's charge. I can't find any legislative history that would suggest for a minute that we're supposed to provide long-term nursing care. It might be that the country is going to want it, but I think the country wants to figure out what it's going to cost them, and they're going to hesitate. But there will be other medical services that will develop.

People, I think, learn very quickly. I think consumers have become educated very quickly in what's available to them, and they make more sophisticated use of services available.

Beneficiary Costs

We will have increased costs. How are we going to pay for that? I really don't know. My own feeling about the Medicare payment system now is that it's not very progressive. I don't like the idea of the $15 that everybody pays regardless of their income, and somehow I'm not sure whether I want to lower the $15 or just make sure that any future increases are spread somewhere along in proportion to people's income. The latter seems somewhat more fair, to me.

I'm concerned about the deductible, the first-day hospital charge which, I gather, is scheduled to go up tremendously in the next year or so, and how that impacts on people.

As I see it, 40 percent of the single women over 65 in this country have only Social Security as income. Sixty percent of black women over 65 have only Social Security as income. The average Social Security payment there is right around $600—$500 for black women, $600 for white women. Unless they've dropped low enough to get into the Medicaid box, a $400 deductible for a first day of hospital care could be a devastating expense. It ought not to be, you know. There ought to be a way to resolve that, and I can't begin to think what we'll do.

The Part B premiums will go up, as sure as God made green apples. There are alternatives. Do we want to reach down? Do we want to raise the Medicare tax for working people to pay for elderly people? It's an option. Do you want a means test? Some of my Republican colleagues have a couple of different approaches to that—taking the actuarial value of the Medicare insurance and adding that to the system the same way we take your income and decide whether to tax your Social Security benefits or not. Another way is to adjust the premium based on income, which, of the two, I think is somewhat fairer.

So there are a lot of options in the future. I think it's an excellent system.

I was interested to find that my own physician in California didn't believe that he ought to take Medicare assignment. He tells me he never felt we would give participating physicians an increase anyway. I know it's because he didn't want those scruffy poor people cluttering up his fancy waiting room. But he's still a nice guy, and he practices in a hospital that has, I guess, less than 1 or 2 percent of what I would call income from low-income people, and, I guess, always will. But I think that we're going to have to make some changes, and with the help of a lot of interested professionals such as yourself, we will.

I think it's one of the more bipartisan subcommittees that I have ever had the privilege to serve with, and I think the people who serve on it genuinely want to work together to produce good legislation.

Medicare Reform and the Federal Budget

As I say, our first job is going to be dealing with the budget cut. We were fortunate in getting some income allocations out of our Budget Committee on the House side, so that it's conceivable we might only have to cut $2.5 billion out of the program, where the Senate is looking for about $4 billion. We're waiting for the House-Senate conference report to see what our mark is going to be, and then we will proceed to write a bill. My hope is that, if we do a bill, we do it this summer because of the other business of the Ways and Means Committee. The tax reform bill—if it doesn't die this summer—will eat up most of September and October.

For those of you who are concerned about what we'll do in regard to the budget, I think you can look for us to act very quickly after we get the indication from the budget conference. Even before it goes to a vote, as soon as we know what the conference committee is going to do, I think we'll begin to move to write a bill.

Discussion

Taxing Employer-Provided Benefits

MS. DARLING: I'd like to get your opinion on the minimum health insurance tax of the administration—"Treasury II."

REP. STARK: The which?

MS. DARLING: The minimum—the floor.

REP. STARK: Oh, on taxing benefits?

MS. DARLING: Yes.

REP. STARK: I want to preface this by saying that I took a pledge some months ago, with many of the other members of the Ways and Means Committee, to the chairman that we would not make a commitment to anybody to take anything off the table in terms of tax reform, whether that's homeowners' mortgage interest or fringe benefit taxation or anything else. We had hoped to keep all those things there as something to review in the process of trying to reform the tax system.

As a person who has a strong, highly organized district that's responsive to labor's concerns, I was surprised that labor seemed to be much more opposed to the $170 cap, as it were, knowing full well that we might get very quickly to $250, which was proposed several times inside the Treasury, and are willing to start taxing on the lowest plans at $10 and $25.

That seems wrong. Just don't isolate that and say that somewhere in the process of tax reform we're going to tax fringe benefits. I would like to stop the growth of tax-free fringe benefits, because they have eroded the tax and FICA [Federal Insurance Contributions Act] base.

That's what Mr. Conable[1] and I tried to do last year when we wrote the fringe benefits bill. We said, let's take the traditional benefits, make them statutory, and not have any more.

We're getting requests every day to add something. Somebody wants free airline passes. Somebody else wants a discount on this or that. And I don't think we can do that. I do think, as a Democrat, that it's the wrong end of the scale.

---

[1]Editor's note: The reference is to Barber Conable, former New York congressman and senior Republican on the House Committee on Ways and Means.

Now the United Auto Workers told me that their people have a benefit package worth $400 a month, and I figure that's got to include a limousine and a driver to take them to their analysis session four times a week. I don't know how you could spend $400 a month on an employee benefit package for health. I buy health insurance from Aetna for my employees for middle-aged people with three and four kids for that amount, and that's paying both sides and with a very small group.

I gather that seems to be more of their concern, because that's their bargaining position, to increase the top end. And if you take the tax deductibility away from that, I guess it's not as attractive. So they seem to be very complacent about the low end, as is Senator Packwood.[2] I'm uncomfortable with that.

MR. SEIDMAN: Your're going to be hearing from Lane Kirkland next week, and you'll find out we are not complacent about the low end. We are opposing the low end, and I've heard him say so.

REP. STARK: Well, I'm glad; because I think that's urgent, and, as I say, if we're going to deal with fringe benefits, it makes no sense to me to single out health. I have always felt we should limit the non-taxability of fringe benefits, but I would include in that life insurance and vacation programs and gymnasiums and parking and airline passes and employee discounts, and the whole schmeer, because in the long run it's counterproductive. I am glad to hear that labor will speak out loudly on that, because it's even worse than in the first proposal.

MS. ELIOPOULOS: Why is it worse?

REP. STARK: Because it's so completely regressive. It impacts so hard on those people with the most minimal plans and, one would presume, the most minimal income. I have people in my district that don't have a $400 paycheck, much less a $400 fringe benefit package. Those are the people that I think we have to be concerned about first.

---

[2]Editor's note: The reference is to Bob Packwood (R-OR), chairman of the Senate Committee on Finance.

Appendix A
Forum Participants

Moderator

Dallas L. Salisbury
Employee Benefit Research
Institute

Speakers

Sheila P. Burke
Office of the Senate Majority
Leader

Cynthia K. Hosay
Martin E. Segal Company

Stephen H. Long
Congressional Budget Office

John C. Rother
American Association of Retired
Persons

Rep. Fortney H. (Pete) Stark
Chairman, Health Subcommittee
Committee on Ways and Means

John F. Troy
The Travelers Insurance
Companies

Karen Williams
Health Insurance Association of
America

Participants

Ken Apfel
Office of Senator Bill Bradley

Paul Berger
Arnold & Porter

Amy Biderman
Health Insurance Association of
America

Elliott Carlson
American Association of Retired
Persons

Thomas P. Cerneka
Tillinghast, Nelson & Warren,
Inc.

Molly Joel Coye
New Jersey Governor's Office of
Policy and Planning

Carol A. Cronin
Washington Business Group on
Health

Helen Darling
Government Research
Corporation

Joe Davidson
The Wall Street Journal

Kathy Deignan
Senate Committee on the Budget

Richard DeLouise
U.S. News & World Report

Dale R. Detlefs
William M. Mercer-Meidinger,
Incorporated

Henry A. DiPrete
John Hancock Mutual Life
Insurance Company

Faye Drummond
Office of Sen. Daniel Moynihan

Phoebe Eliopoulos
Benefits Today, BNA

Marilyn Falik
CIGNA Corporation

Mary Jane Fisher
National Underwriter

Theresa Forster
Office of Sen. David Pryor

Beth Fuchs
Senate Special Committee on
Aging

Kathleen Gardner-Cravedi
Subcommittee on Health and
  Long-Term Care, House Select
  Committee on Aging

William E. Giegerich
Buck Consultants, Inc.

Aileen Goldberg
Health Care Publications

Marian Gornick
Health Care Financing
  Administration

Judy Haberek
Washington Health Costs Letter

Bill Halamandaris
Foundation for Hospice and
  Home Care

Donald P. Harrington
AT&T

Howard Hennington
Mutual of America Life
  Insurance Company

Robert T. Hollinshead
National Rural Electric
  Cooperative Association

Michael Hoon
Office of Sen. Malcolm Wallop

Paul H. Jackson
The Wyatt Company

John B. Keenan
IU International Management
  Corp.

Kenneth K. Keene
Johnson & Higgins

Kerry Kilpatrick
Office of Sen. Dave Durenberger

John K. Kittredge
The Prudential Insurance
  Company of America

Nicholas D. Latrenta
Metropolitan Life Insurance
  Company

C. William Lee
E. I. duPont de Nemours &
  Company, Inc.

Marvin A. Levins
Connecticut General Life
  Insurance Company

Marion Ein Lewin
American Enterprise Institute

John F. McCaffrey
Frank B. Hall Consulting
  Company

Kathy McCarl
The Equitable Life Assurance
  Society of the United States

Stephen McConnell
Senate Special Committee on
  Aging

Richard W. McLaughlin
The Travelers Insurance
  Companies

Jeffrey C. Merrill
The Robert Wood Johnson
  Foundation

Clay Mickel
American Hospital Association

Curtis Mikkelsen
Morgan Guaranty Trust
  Company of New York

Marilyn Moon
The Urban Institute

Warren L. Moser
Southwestern Bell Telephone
  Company

Mary Mundinger
Senate Committee on Labor &
  Human Resources

Janet Myder
National Council of Senior
  Citizens

Patricia Neuman
Johns Hopkins University

106

Robert D. Paul
Martin E. Segal Company

Mark Pauly
The Leonard Davis Institute
University of Pennsylvania

Marla Posner
Changing Times

Melvyn J. Rodrigues
Atlantic Richfield Company

Shannon Salmon
Senate Committee on Finance

John C. Scioli
New Jersey Department of
　Health

Bert Seidman
AFL-CIO

Kenneth P. Shapiro
Hay/Huggins Company, Inc.

Harry Smith
Sun Company, Inc.

Quentin I. Smith
Towers, Perrin, Forster &
　Crosby, Inc.

Katherine Bauer Somers
National Academy of Sciences

Joseph Stahl
Towers, Perrin, Forster &
　Crosby, Inc.

Stephen Somers
The Robert Wood Johnson
　Foundation

Wendy Weisbrod
Office of Rep. Lawrence Smith

Raymond L. Willis
United Technologies Corporation

Leah R. Young
Journal of Commerce

EBRI Staff

Emily S. Andrews
Director of Research

Deborah J. Chollet
Research Associate

Robert B. Friedland
Research Associate

Jeannette Hahm
Research Assistant and
　Computer Programmer

Sophie M. Korczyk
Research Associate

Anne L. Mayberry
Education & Communications
　Associate

Frank B. McArdle
Director, Education and
　Communications

Bonnie Newton
Education & Communications
　Associate

Joseph S. Piacentini
Research Assistant

Stephanie L. Poe
Education & Communications
　Associate

Lisa A. Schenkel
Education & Communications
　Associate

Mona Seliger
Research Assistant

Appendix B
Medicare Benefits and Financing: Report of the 1982 Advisory Council on Social Security

(Following is the "Executive Summary of Recommendations" from the report.)

The Advisory Council on Social Security, appointed in September of 1982, was requested to focus its attention on Title XVIII of the Social Security Act, the Federal Hospital Insurance (HI) and the Federal Supplementary Medical Insurance (SMI) programs. The appointment of the National Commission on Social Security Reform to address the fiscal problems of the Old Age and Survivors Insurance (OASI) and Disability Insurance (DI) programs precluded the need for this Council to undertake an in-depth review of those programs.

Over the past 15 months, the Council reviewed both the HI (Part A) and SMI (Part B) programs of Medicare and the status of their respective trust funds. Because of the serious financial problems projected for the Hospital Insurance Trust Fund, principal attention was devoted to the Part A. The majority of the Council's recommendations address this part of Medicare.

The Council's recommendations were designed to accomplish two objectives: first, to provide a means for maintaining the fiscal integrity of the Hospital Insurance Trust Fund through 1995; and second, to provide improvements in the manner in which health care is financed and delivered which will alleviate some of the financial pressures on the trust fund in the future.

The Council adopted the following summary resolution:

> The Council acknowledges a probable deficit in the Hospital Insurance trust fund in 1995 by an amount between $200- and $300 billion, depending upon the optimistic or pessimistic view of the price changes in the medical industry and the economy generally in the next few years. The Council believes that the savings identified in its recommendations concerning Medicare eligibility, reimbursement, and benefit structure will account for a substantial portion of this anticipated deficit. The Council further believes the recommendations on anticipated sources of revenues from taxation of a portion of employer-provided health benefits, the alcohol and tobacco taxes, and, if required, the reallocation

of payroll taxes to the HI trust fund, will be sufficient to cover additional funding needs through 1995.[1]

The Council's recommendations addressed issues of program financing, eligibility, benefit structure, reimbursement, and several issues considered general in nature.

Program Financing Recommendations:

- *The Advisory Council on Social Security believes that the most critical problem facing the Medicare program—in both the short- and long-range— is the projected insolvency of the Hospital Insurance trust fund. Anticipated outlays in excess of income are expected to deplete this fund before the end of the 1980s.* The Council recommends that planning for the financial stability of the Hospital Insurance trust fund should recognize the likelihood of a $200 to $300 billion deficit in this fund by the year 1995.* (Chapter II, A.)

- *The Advisory Council on Social Security opposes any increase in the use of general revenues to finance the Medicare Hospital Insurance trust fund.*

  The Council questions the soundness of any policy which relies upon general revenues to finance the HI program. In an era when the government is experiencing substantial annual deficits, reliance on general revenues would only serve to exacerbate the problem of increasing deficits. (Chapter II, B.)

- *The Advisory Council opposes any further increase in scheduled HI payroll taxes.*

  A substantial majority of Council members oppose raising revenues through an increase in payroll taxes because of the potentially adverse effects such taxes would have on employment and business activity. The Council believed that a tax which is not progressive unduly burdens middle- and low-income workers. The current payroll tax already imposes a substantial burden on such workers and should not be increased. (Chapter II, C.)

---

[1]The most recent estimates of the HCFA Actuary, information received subsequent to the Council's concluding meeting, reflect that if moderate economic assumptions, i.e., Alternative IIB, prevail the 1995 deficit, considering only the amount that expenditures will exceed revenues, will be $156.3 billion. When a reserve equal to 50 percent of expected expenditures is included, the total shortfall in the trust fund will be $225 to $235 billion. (The Board of Trustees of the HI trust fund has adopted the general financing principle that there should be a reserve in the trust fund equal to one-half of a year's disbursements.) Obviously, if the more pessimistic assumptions materialize this deficit figure will be greater. All Council votes and recommendations were predicated on cumulative deficit and reserve requirements of up to $300 billion in 1995.

*Predicated on present law, funding and expenditure control policies, beneficiary entitlement changes and other policies.

- *The Council believes that the individuality of the Old Age and Survivors Insurance, Disability Insurance and Hospital Insurance programs should be maintained, and that each program should be funded at a level sufficient to meet its continuing needs. Where short-term interfund borrowing among the trust funds is deemed necessary, such borrowing should be subject to appropriate safeguards which include authority for each fund to borrow from the others, specific repayment schedules and prohibition against reducing the lending fund's assets below an actuarially acceptable level.*

The Council recognizes that interfund borrowing has been used in the past and now has been reauthorized through 1987. However, the Council was pleased that legislation enacted in 1983 that reauthorized such interfund borrowing included provisions that address the Council's concerns. (Chapter II, D.)

- *The Council recommends that, if needed, consideration be given to a reallocation of payroll tax rates between OASDI and HI in order to transfer sufficient OASDI surplus revenues to HI during the period 1985 through 1995 to maintain the financial viability of the HI trust fund.*

The Council believes that the diversion of projected surplus OASDI revenues by a reallocation of contribution rates among the OASI, DI and HI trust funds is a viable method for alleviating a substantial portion of the short-term projected HI deficit. However, the Council recognizes that both long- and short-range considerations must govern any specific reallocation proposal. Reallocation should only be considered if the integrity of all three trust funds will be preserved. (Chapter II, E.)

- *The Council endorses the Administration's proposal to consider any employer's contribution to an employee's health benefit plan that exceeds $70 a month for an individual and $175 a month for a family as income to the employee and subject to Federal, State and local taxes in the same manner as wages.*

The Council also recommends that consideration should be given to earmarking an appropriate portion of the incremental revenues that would be realized from the proposed tax to Medicare's Hospital Insurance trust fund.

A substantial majority of Council members believes that the principal benefit to be derived from this tax exempt limitation is that it will bring about a change in consumer health care purchasing patterns by increasing consumer cost consciousness and provider competitiveness that will slow the increase in health care costs. Removing the current complete tax exemption of these benefits will make employees more conscious of and concerned about the cost of health care and the cost effectiveness of the services they receive.

Revenue-raising possibilities under this recommendation were a secondary consideration. (Chapter II, F.)

- *The Council recommends that Federal excise taxes on alcohol and tobacco be increased, with the increased revenue to be earmarked to the HI trust fund. The Council does not specify the amount to be raised and earmarked, but suggests that the amount be determined by the Congress.*

111

Although the Advisory Council generally views increased taxes as an undesirable alternative for resolving the financial problem facing the hospital insurance trust fund, the projected substantial deficit precludes a resolution based solely on a reduction of expenditures. A majority of Council members recommend an increase in the Federal excise tax on alcohol and tobacco products based on the demonstrated correlation between the use of these products and increased health care costs. (Chapter II, G).

Program Eligibility Recommendations:

- *The Council recommends an increase in the age of eligibility for Medicare benefits from age 65 to 67. This recommendation provides for the age of eligibility to be increased by three-month increments per year beginning on January 1, 1985. Beginning on January 1, 1989, the rate of increase will escalate to six-month increments, achieving full implementation of the age 67 eligibility on January 1, 1990. The Council further recommends that, subsequently, the age of eligibility for Medicare benefits should be indexed to increases in life expectancy.*

A majority of the Council members concluded that the age of 65 as the initial age of eligibility was rooted more in custom than on assessment of health care needs. The age of eligibility for unreduced monthly social security retirement benefits has been increased to age 67 although full implementation of the new age will not occur until the third decade of the 21st century. However, there is no inherent linkage between eligibility for monthly retirement benefits and Medicare as today more than 50 percent of those eligible for social security elect reduced old age benefits up to 3 years prior to the age at which they may first become eligible for Medicare.

Recognizing the increase in life expectancy since 1966, the year of Medicare's enactment, and the increased cost of health care services to those of advancing years, the Council believes it is necessary to assure that Medicare's resources are focused on the population most in need of Medicare protection. A substantial majority of the Council conclude that there is a need to adjust the age of eligibility to reflect the changes in life expectancy that have already occurred and to accomplish this adjustment by the end of the decade. With respect to the future, the Council recommends periodic adjustments to reflect changes in life expectancy. (Chapter III, A.)

- *The Council concurs with the recommendations of the National Commission on Social Security Reform and with subsequently enacted provisions of Public Law 98-21, that provide (1) that Old Age, Survivors, Disability and Hospital Insurance (OASDHI) coverage be extended on a mandatory basis to employees of nonprofit organizations, and (2) that State and local government units which have elected OASDHI coverage for their employees be precluded from terminating such coverage in the future, including termination actions underway but not completed by the April 20, 1983 date of enactment of Public Law 98-21.*

112

The Council concludes that coverage under Medicare of all persons in paid employment is a desirable objective that would contribute to the fiscal stability of the OASI, DI and HI programs. Therefore, the Council believes that the recent enactment of provisions mandating coverage for all employees of nonprofit organizations and precluding terminations of coverage by State and local employees along with prior legislative action covering all current and future Federal workers under the HI program has contributed to this objective. (Chapter II, B.)

- *The Council opposes any further extension of Medicare coverage to individuals (not otherwise eligible based on age or disability status) on the basis of medical diagnosis or the medical necessity for a particular form of treatment. Should specific categories of disease be considered in the future for Federal financial assistance, such assistance should be provided through a special program with separate allocation of funds to pay for the required treatment.*

The Council acknowledges the success of the End Stage Renal Disease (ESRD) provisions of Medicare, enacted in 1972, in providing financial assistance to those in need of this expensive treatment. However, the Council believes that in the future, the Medicare program's eligibility requirement should be restricted to existing beneficiary categories i.e., aged and disabled, and any special disease categories requiring financial assistance should be separately funded. (Chapter III, C.)

Benefit Structure Recommendations:

- *The Council recommends a restructuring of the Medicare Part A Hospital Insurance program to provide:*

1. Unlimited hospital inpatient days per calendar year.

2. A per admission deductible, as currently computed, but limited to two hospital admissions per calendar year.

3. A daily coinsurance, equal to 3 percent of the hospital inpatient deductible, for all inpatient days except the initial day of any stay where an inpatient deductible applies.

4. A skilled nursing facility benefit of 100 days per calendar year with no coinsurance on days 1 through 20 and a 12.5 percent coinsurance on days 21–100.

5. The current home health benefit.

6. The current hospice benefit.

The Council recommends an enhanced Part A Hospital Insurance benefit be offered to beneficiaries as an integral part of their Part B (SMI) election that provides for:

1. Elimination of the 3 percent daily coinsurance on hospital inpatient days.

2. Elimination of the 12.5 percent daily coinsurance on days 21–100 of skilled nursing facility stay benefits.

If a beneficiary elects to take Medicare's Part B coverage he/she automatically elects the Part A enhanced benefit. The enhanced Part A benefit would be financed with an actuarially sound premium. This premium would include an additional amount for the purpose of providing additional revenues necessary to help to resolve the current disparity between beneficiary contributions to the HI trust fund and the value of benefits received.

The Council also recommends an enhanced Part B benefit to be offered on an optional basis, i.e., not as an integral part of the beneficiary's Part B election. The enhanced benefit would provide a yearly limit on Part B out-of-pocket expenses, which would be indexed annually to recognize increases in per capita Part B program expenditures. The Part B option would also be financed by a premium which would be added to the current Part B premium for those electing this option. (See recommendation #16.)

The Council concludes that while the hospital insurance program of Medicare, Part A, provides adequate coverage for most beneficiaries, it does not provide adequate protection in the event of catastrophic illness. The Council believes that financing an improved benefit package for all Medicare beneficiaries through increased coinsurances on shorter hospital stays would place the financial burden only on those who were ill and required inpatient care. The establishment of a premium to finance improved benefits and to generate additional revenues to help insure the fiscal soundness of the program is a more equitable means of sharing additional beneficiary costs.

The Council believes that the changes it is recommending will also facilitate beneficiary understanding of their benefits under Medicare and simplify administration of the program.

Recognizing beneficiary concerns regarding increasing cost-sharing liability under the Part B supplementary medical insurance program, the Council concludes that offering, on an optional basis, the opportunity to limit cost-sharing liability for Part B services to an annual dollar amount would improve the protection available and preclude or reduce the need to purchase private supplemental insurance.

Although the Council recognizes that the recommended restructured benefit package will increase beneficiary contributions under the Medicare program the benefits offered will be improved and at less cost than comparable Medicare/Medigap protection. (Chapter IV, A.)

• *The Council recommends that the Secretary of Health and Human Services, in developing a comprehensive long term care program, seek guidance from those studies which have suggested the targeting of groups who will benefit from these services.*

The Council recognizes the problems faced by the Medicare population due to the fragmentation among several programs of services offered to beneficiaries who need ongoing chronic care. As the Medicare population

114

ages, the Council believes that the need for long term care services will increase.

The Council believes that more conclusive information regarding the long term care needs of the elderly is needed. Recognizing the potentially high cost of such care, any expansion of long term care benefits under the Medicare program, especially at a time when the program is experiencing serious fiscal problems, would not be appropriate. A piecemeal attack on the critical problem of financing long term care will not work. Development of a comprehensive program is necessary. Any long term care program should target those who are eligible for conventional long term care and provide alternative care as a substitute for more expensive conventional care. (Chapter IV, B.)

- *The Council believes, in general, that the elderly can benefit from prevention-oriented programs and screening procedures. The Council suggests that a comprehensive review of the Health Care Financing Administration's demonstration projects to assess the economy and efficacy of expanding Medicare coverage to include preventive services be undertaken prior to any change in the law.*

The Council views as inconclusive the evidence concerning the cost-effectiveness of preventive services. The offering of such services may improve health and mobility of the elderly and produce long-term program savings. However, while there was agreement that there must be preventive services that could be shown to be cost-effective, a comprehensive study should be undertaken to identify those particular services before expansion of Medicare's coverage of preventive care. (Chapter IV, C.)

- *The Council recommends the use of a voluntary voucher in the Medicare program. The voucher would provide beneficiaries with an alternative to the current method of reimbursing medical services. The voucher would also promote the development of more efficient ways of delivering services by health care providers.*

The Council is in general agreement that a voucher system represents one means for the promotion of competition in the health industry and that such a system would increase incentives for beneficiaries to be more sensitive to the cost of health care services. Although the Council opposes any mandatory voucher system, a substantial majority support a voluntary system provided beneficiaries are given adequate assistance in the process of choosing an alternative health care plan. (Chapter IV. D.)

- *The Council recommends that the current Supplementary Medical Insurance (Part B) deductible be indexed to the Consumer Price Index (CPI) to keep pace with inflation and with increases in beneficiary income. The indexing should begin as soon as feasible.*

Unlike the inpatient deductible under the Part A Hospital Insurance program which is indexed to the cost of hospital care, increases in the Part B supplementary medical insurance deductible are adjusted periodically by Congress. The Council believes that increases that have been

115

legislated have failed to keep pace with either the increasing cost of Part B services or the increasing income available to the elderly.

Given the historic greater increase in the cost of medical services, the Council acknowledges that indexing the deductible to medical costs could produce a disparity between income increases and deductible increases over time. The Council, therefore, recommends that the Part B deductible be indexed to the Consumer Price index as soon as feasible to insure a more reasonable ratio between beneficiary income and Part B cost sharing. (Chapter IV, E.)

Program Reimbursement Recommendations:

- *The Council endorses the principle of prospective payment for Medicare inpatient hospital services. The Council supports a prospective payment system based on diagnosis provided it is equitable for all hospitals, encourages efficiency of operations and maintains accessibility and quality of care for Medicare beneficiaries.*

  The Council recognizes that the allowed rate of increase in the DRG rates will have a significant impact upon the costs of the Medicare hospital insurance program. Therefore, the Council urges the Secretary of HHS to exert care to limit any annual rate of growth in the DRG rates that is above the annual rate of change in the hospital input price index. (Chapter V, A.)

- *The Council believes that it is inappropriate for the Medicare program, which is designed to pay for medical services provided to the elderly, to underwrite the cost of training medical personnel and recommends that such support be withdrawn as alternative funding sources are identified. The Council believes that medical education is an appropriate area for governmental support and recommends that the Department of Health and Human Services undertake a study to identify and develop other Federal, State, and local funding sources.* (Chapter V, B.)

- *The Council believes that Medicare's statutorily mandated reasonable charge method of reimbursement has not been effective in controlling expenditures or encouraging utilization of cost effective services. As a step toward reform of the system, the Council recommends a statutory revision to authorize reimbursement based on fee schedules adjusted initially and periodically for differences in cost of living and/or maintaining a practice. The Council urges that development of the schedules be undertaken with due concern for all interested parties, direct input from the medical profession, and with maintenance of support for the capitation system.*

  The Council believes that the current reasonable charge system has failed to curb inflation in medical care costs and, in fact, has probably contributed to that inflation. The current system has also helped to perpetuate significant payment differentials among geographic areas and medical specialties. The Council views fee schedules as the initial step in reform of the system and encourages the medical profession and other third party payors to cooperate in experimenting with and developing alternative methods of reimbursement. (Chapter V, C.)

116

- *The Council recommends a statutory revision to the current Medicare assignment system. The revision would establish a physician participation agreement system under which physicians would annually elect whether they would "participate," i.e., accept assignment on all services to Medicare patients. Notice of intent to participate, or to withdraw from participation, would be made six months in advance. Claims for reimbursement for services furnished by physicians who decided not to participate would always be unassigned, and program payment would always be made to the patient who would be responsible for the physician's entire bill including any amount that exceeds Medicare's reasonable charge.*

  The Council recommends the following incentives for physicians to participate:

  —*Competition: The Medicare program would publish annually a directory of participating physicians. The directory would be published on a local basis, e.g., city, county or Standard Metropolitan Statistical Area (SMSA), as appropriate.*

  —*Billing: Participating physicians could take advantage of streamlined billing and payment procedures. Such incentives could include provisions for multiple-list claims, automated or electronic billing with the program providing some of the necessary equipment and an electronic funds transfer (EFT) process.* (Chapter V, D.)

General Recommendations:

- *The Council recommends that it should be a fundamental policy of the Department of Health and Human Services to promote the development of medical technology. Criteria used to evaluate new technology should stress the efficacy of new procedures as well as their cost.*

  The Council believes that the development of new medical technology and procedures should be encouraged. At the same time the Council believes that greater attention must be given to the criteria used to evaluate new technology. The initial cost of new technology is one criterion for assessment. Lower cost, brought about by economies of scale, is another criterion. Value, however, is a criterion of no less importance. It must be measured by the benefit that new technology brings to medicine itself, to international competitiveness for the United States and, most of all, to the healthful lives of the American people. (Chapter VI, A.)

- *The Council supports the concept of voluntary advance directives as a means of appropriate decision-making about life-sustaining treatment for incapacitated patients. Also, recognizing that this is an individual State determination, the Council encourages a voluntary program in the 14 States where advanced directives are legal and encourages the other 36 State legislatures to enact such legislation. In the States where this is legal, the Council suggests that a person be offered a living will when he/she applies for Medicare.*

  The Council further suggests that the guidelines employed for this voluntary program be those found in the report on "Deciding to Forego Life-Sustaining

Treatment" by the President's Commission for the Study of Ethical Problems in Medicine and Biomedical and Behavioral Research.

The Council recommends HCFA undertake a comparative study to assess what the impacts (financial and otherwise) have been in those 14 States that have living wills compared to those States without them. (Chapter VI, B.)

- The Council recommends that the Health Care Financing Administration continue its efforts to improve the management of the Medicare program. As part of this effort, HCFA should review the recommendations of the President's Private Sector Survey on Cost Control and the Office of the Inspector General of the Department of Health and Human Services.

The Council believes that if the American people are to be asked to make sacrifices to preserve the financial viability of the Medicare program, they must be assured that program managers are striving to contain the cost of the Medicare program and assure that it will carry out its mission to make first class health care available to the elderly and disabled of this country. (Chapter VI, C.)

- *The Council opposes any effort to tie entitlement to Medicare benefits to a beneficiary's financial status.*

The Council rejects the concept of "means testing," believing that Medicare should remain an entitlement program where individual income or wealth is not a factor considered in determining one's eligibility for benefits. (Chapter VI, D.)

The Council recommends further study of three additional program issues:

1. Proposals for long term restructure of the Medicare program which encourage individuals to save during working years for the purpose of purchasing health care coverage in retirement years. Such proposals could establish universal individual "health credit accounts" and further encourage savings through tax deductible accounts similar to individual retirement accounts (IRAs). Medicare would be modified to complement individual spending during retirement years. (Chapter VII A and B.)

2. Improvement of Medicare's current program of information and assistance to beneficiaries. This effort should be a joint undertaking between the Health Care Financing Administration and the Social Security Administration. (Chapter VII, C.)

3. Identification of additional areas where Medicare could serve as a secondary payor to the group health insurance for the working aged or their spouses. The study would include evaluation of implementation of current provisions and consideration of appropriate areas in which to expand the concept. (Chapter VII, D.)

The Council views these issues, particularly the long range restructure concept, as deserving of further study and evaluation.

Appendix C
Summary of 1985 Annual Reports of the Medicare Board of Trustees

Introduction

This summary presents an overview of the information contained in the annual reports of the trustees required under Title XVIII of the Social Security Act, Health Insurance for the Aged and Disabled, commonly known as Medicare. There are two basic programs under Medicare:

(1) Hospital Insurance (HI) which pays for inpatient hospital care and other related care of those aged 65 and over and of the long-term disabled; and

(2) Supplementary Medical Insurance (SMI) which pays for physicians' services, outpatient hospital services and other medical expenses of those aged 65 and over and of the long-term disabled.

The HI program is financed primarily by payroll taxes, with the taxes paid by current workers used primarily to pay benefits to current beneficiaries. However, the HI program maintains a trust fund to provide a small reserve against fluctuations and to anticipate changes in the demographic makeup of the population. The SMI program is financed on an accrual basis with a contingency margin. This means that the SMI trust fund should always be somewhat greater than the claims that have been incurred by enrollees but not yet paid by the program. The trust funds hold all of the income not currently needed to pay benefits and related expenses. The assets of the funds may not be used for any other purpose; however, they may be invested in certain interest-bearing obligations of the U.S. Government.

The secretaries of Treasury, Labor, Health and Human Services, and two public members serve as trustees of the HI and SMI trust funds. The Secretary of Treasury is the managing trustee. The administrator of the Health Care Financing Administration, the agency charged with administering the Medicare program, is the secretary of the Board of Trustees.

Copies of the complete 1985 HI and SMI annual reports can be obtained from the Health Care Financing Administration, Office of Public Affairs, Room 658 East High Rise, 6325 Security Blvd., Baltimore, MD 21235.

Hospital Insurance Trust Fund

As mentioned in the introduction, the HI trust fund is financed primarily by payroll taxes. The HI contribution rates applicable to taxable earnings in each of the calendar years 1983 and later are shown in table 1. The maximum taxable amounts of annual earnings are shown for 1983 through 1985. After 1985, the automatic increase provisions in section 230 of the Social Security Act determine the maximum taxable amount.

TABLE 1
Contribution Rates and Maximum Taxable Amount of Annual Earnings

Calendar Year	Maximum Taxable Amount of Annual Earnings	Contribution Rate (Percent of Taxable Earnings)	
		Employees and Employers, Each	Self-Employed
1983	35,700	1.30	1.30
1984	37,800	1.30	2.60
1985	39,600	1.35	2.70

Changes scheduled in present law:

1986 & later	Subject to automatic increase	1.45	2.90

The Social Security Act was amended during 1984. The major provisions among the many affecting the HI program are:

(1) The Medicare secondary payor provision for workers and their spouses aged 65 to 69 who are covered by an employer's group health insurance is extended to cases where the employee has not reached age 65 and has a spouse age 65 through 69. Effective January 1, 1985.

(2) The increase for hospital payments in fiscal year 1985 is equal to the increase in the hospital input price index (the cost of the mix of goods and services used to provide inpatient hospital services) plus one quarter of one percent. However, budget neutrality continues to apply in fiscal year 1985. In fiscal year 1986, the rate of increase cannot exceed the increase in the hospital input price index plus one quarter of one percent.

(3) Reimbursement for capital upon the change of ownership of a hospital or skilled nursing facility is restricted to the lesser of the cost under

120

Medicare to the owner of record (on July 18, 1984) or the purchase price. The costs of legal fees, negotiations, or settlement of the sale are no longer reimbursable. The recapture of depreciation up to the full value of the initial asset under Medicare is required.

(4) Durable medical equipment provided by home health agencies as part of a covered home health service will no longer be reimbursed at 100 percent of cost. Reimbursement will be at no more than 60 percent of reasonable cost and the beneficiary will be responsible for a 20 percent coinsurance payment. Effective upon enactment.

Operations of the HI Program—In calendar year 1984, about 27 million people over age 65 and almost three million disabled people under age 65 were covered under HI, financed primarily by the contributions of 122 million workers through payroll taxes. Payroll taxes during 1984 amounted to $42.3 billion, accounting for 90.5 percent of all HI income. About 2.1 percent of all income resulted from a lump sum transfer from the general fund of the Treasury for military service wage credits, and reimbursements for benefits for certain uninsured persons. Interest payments to the HI fund amounted to 6.5 percent of all HI income for 1984. The remaining 0.8 percent was contributed through premiums paid by voluntary enrollees and taxes collected from railroad workers. Of the $43.9 billion in HI disbursements, $43.3 billion was for benefit payments while the remaining $0.6 billion was spent for administrative expenses. HI administrative expenses were 1.4 percent of total disbursements.

Table 2 displays the HI fund operations for calendar years 1978–1984. In most years, the HI fund has increased. However, the fund ratio (the fund at the beginning of the year divided by disbursements during the year) has declined every year from 1979 to 1981. The fund ratio increased slightly at the beginning of 1982, primarily due to the increase in the contribution rate in 1981. The fund ratio dropped dramatically at the beginning of 1983, primarily due to the interfund loan made to the OASI trust fund.

Actuarial Status of the Trust Fund—The Board of Trustees has adopted the general financing principle that annual income to the hospital insurance program should be at least equal to annual outlays of the program plus an amount to maintain a balance in the trust fund equal to a minimum of one-half year's disbursements. At the beginning of 1985, the trust fund was far below this desired level. Projections were made under four alternative sets of assumptions: optimistic, two intermediate sets (alternatives II-A and II-B), and pessimistic. Under both sets of intermediate assumptions, the trust fund ratio is

121

TABLE 2
HI Fund Operations Calendar Years 1978–1984
(Amounts in Billions)

Calendar Year	Total Income	Total Disbursements	Interfund Borrowing Transfers	Net Increase in Fund	Fund at End of Year	Ratio at Beginning of Year
1978	$19.2	$18.2		$ 1.0	$11.5	57%
1979	22.8	21.1		1.8	13.2	54
1980	26.1	25.6		0.5	13.7	52
1981	35.7	30.7		5.0	18.7	45
1982	38.0	36.1	$ − 12.4	− 10.6	8.2	52
1983	44.6	39.9		− 4.7	12.9	21
1984	46.7	43.9		− 2.8	15.7	29

Note: Components may not add to totals due to rounding.

projected to increase until about 1990 and then decline steadily until the fund is completely exhausted in the late 1990s.

Under the more optimistic set of assumptions (alternative I), the trust fund is projected to grow steadily throughout the first 25-year projection period. Under the more pessimistic set of assumptions (alternative III), the trust fund is projected to increase to a level of about 43 percent in 1989 and then decrease rapidly until the fund is exhausted in 1992.

Table 3 summarizes the estimated operations of the HI trust fund under the four alternative sets of assumptions. Figure 1 shows historic trust fund ratios for recent years and projected ratios under the four sets of assumptions.

The adequacy of the financing of the HI program on a long-range basis is measured by comparing on a year-by-year basis the actual tax rates specified by law with the corresponding total costs of the program, expressed as percentages of taxable payroll. The actuarial balance is defined to be the excess of the average tax for the valuation period over the average cost of the program expressed as a percent of taxable payroll. Table 4 compares the actuarial balance under each of the four sets of assumptions for the 75-year projection period 1985–2059. Figure 2 shows the year-by-year costs as a percent of taxable payroll for each of the four sets of assumptions, as well as the scheduled tax rates. The cost figures in table 4 and figure 2 include amounts for building and maintaining the trust fund at the level of a half

FIGURE 1
Short Term HI Trust Fund Ratios

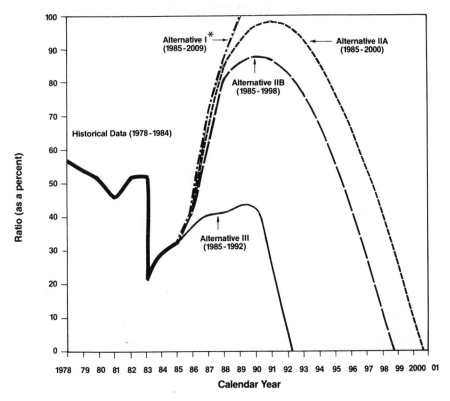

*The trust fund ratio remains over 100 percent under alternative 1 during this 25-year projection period.

Note: The trust fund ratio is defined as the ratio of assets in the trust fund at the beginning of the year to disbursements during the year.

year's disbursements as recommended by the Board of Trustees. Figure 2 emphasizes the inadequacy of the financing of the HI program by illustrating the divergence of the program costs and scheduled tax rates under each set of assumptions. Table 5 presents a comparison of the projected experience in the 1984 and 1985 reports.

Conclusion—Two actions favorably affecting the financial status of the Hospital Insurance Trust Fund have occurred since the pub-

125

TABLE 4
75-Year Actuarial Balance of the Hospital Insurance
Program Under Alternative Sets of Assumptions

	Alternative			
	I	II-A	II-B	III
1985–2009:				
Average contribution rate[1]	2.89%	2.89%	2.89%	2.89%
Average cost of the program[2]	2.85	3.41	3.57	4.86
Actuarial balance	+0.04	−0.52	−0.68	−1.97
2010–2034:				
Average contribution rate[1]	2.90	2.90	2.90	2.90
Average cost of the program[2]	3.17	5.45	5.89	11.66
Actuarial balance	−0.28	−2.55	−2.99	−8.76
2035–2059:				
Average contribution rate[1]	2.90	2.90	2.90	2.90
Average cost of the program[2]	3.83	7.05	7.62	16.10
Actuarial balance	−0.93	−4.15	−4.72	−13.20
1985–2059:				
Average contribution rate[1]	2.90	2.90	2.90	2.90
Average cost of the program[2]	3.28	5.30	5.69	10.87
Actuarial balance	−0.38	−2.40	−2.79	−7.97

[1]As scheduled under present law.
[2]Expressed as a percent of taxable payroll. Includes amounts for trust fund building and maintenance.
Note: Taxable payroll is adjusted to take into account the lower contribution rates on tips and on multiple-employer "excess wages," as compared with the combined employer-employee rate.

lication of the 1984 report. First, the Secretary of Health and Human Services has tentatively decided to set the fiscal year 1986 hospital payment rates at the same level as the fiscal year 1985 rates. Second, legislation has been enacted reducing the annual increase in the rates which can be granted without specific justification from one percent plus the increase in the hospital input price index to one quarter of one percent plus the increase in the hospital price index. Nevertheless, the present financing schedule for the hospital insurance program is barely sufficient to ensure the payment of benefits and maintain the fund at a level of one half year's disbursements over the next 10 to 12 years if the assumptions underlying the estimates are realized. The trust fund is exhausted in the late 1990s under both alternatives

TABLE 5
Status of the Hospital Insurance Trust Fund

Alternative Assumptions	Year in Which the Trust Fund is Exhausted as Published in the		25-Year Actuarial Balance of the HI Program[1] as Published in the		75-Year Actuarial Balance of the HI Program as Published in the 1985 Report
	1984 Report	1985 Report	1984 Report	1985 Report	
I (Optimistic)	1995	[2]	-0.44%	+0.04%	-0.38%
II-A (Intermediate)	1991	2000	-1.24	-0.52	-2.40
II-B (Intermediate)	1991	1998	-1.37	-0.68	-2.79
III (Pessimistic)	1989	1992	-2.71	-1.97	-7.97

[1]The actuarial balance of the hospital insurance program is defined to be the excess of the average tax rate for the valuation period over the average cost of the program, expressed as a percent of taxable payroll, for the same period.
[2]The trust fund is solvent at least through the end of the first 25-year projection period.

FIGURE 2
Estimated HI Cost and Tax Rates

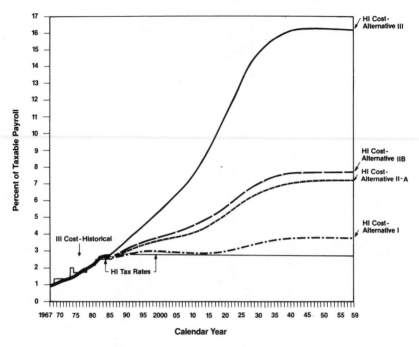

Note: HI projected cost includes an allowance for building and maintaining the trust fund balance at the level of a half-year's outgo after accounting for the offsetting effect of interest earnings.

II-A and II-B. Under the more pessimistic assumptions, the fund is exhausted in 1992. Under the more optimistic alternative I, the trust fund is solvent at least through the first 25-year projection period. In order to bring the hospital insurance program into close actuarial balance for the first 25-year projection period under alternative II-B assumptions, either disbursements of the program will have to be reduced by 19 percent or income will have to be increased by 24 percent.

There are currently over four covered workers supporting each HI enrollee. By the middle of the next century, there will be only slightly more than two covered workers supporting each enrollee. Thus, it will be necessary to build a reserve to finance the program when current workers retire during the first half of the next century. Not only does the projected rate of growth in the program during the next

128

several decades not allow for the building of the necessary reserve, but it results in the depletion of the fund during the late 1990s. Thus, current workers who retire in the next century will not only have to compensate for the shortfall due to high current outlays, but will also derive significantly fewer benefits from their contributions because of the shift in the demographic makeup of the population.

The Board recommends that Congress take further action to curtail the rate of growth in the hospital insurance program in order to increase equity among different generations of beneficiaries and covered workers.

Supplementary Medical Insurance Trust Fund

Financing for the supplementary medical insurance program is established annually on the basis of standard monthly premium rates (paid by or on behalf of all participants) and monthly actuarial rates determined separately for aged and disabled beneficiaries (on which general revenue contributions are based). Prior to the six-month transition period (July 1, 1983 through December 31, 1983) these rates were applicable to the 12-month periods ending June 30. Beginning January 1, 1984, the annual basis was changed to calendar years. Monthly actuarial rates are equal to one-half the monthly amounts necessary to finance the SMI program. These rates determine the amount to be contributed from general revenues on behalf of each enrollee. Based on the formula in the law, the government contribution effectively makes up the difference between twice the monthly actuarial rates and the standard monthly premium rate. Figure 3 presents these values for financing periods since 1974. The extent to which general revenue financing is becoming the major source of income for the program is clearly indicated in this figure.

Standard monthly premium rates and monthly actuarial rates have been announced for periods through December 31, 1985. For calendar year 1985, the standard monthly premium rate is $15.50, and the monthly actuarial rates are $31.00 and $52.70 for the aged and disabled, respectively.

The Social Security Act was amended during 1984. The major provisions among those affecting the SMI program were:

(1) The monthly premium rate for calendar years 1986 and 1987 will be set at one-half the actuarial rate for aged enrollees. In addition, the dollar increase in the SMI premium may not exceed the dollar amount of the Social Security COLA.

(2) For the 15-month period beginning July 1, 1984, physician customary and prevailing charges are frozen/at the levels in effect for the 12-month period ending June 30, 1984. In addition, a participating physician system, whereby physicians may voluntarily agree to accept assignment for all services to Medicare patients, is established. During the freeze period, participating physicians are allowed normal increases in their actual charges, and these increases will be reflected in future customary charges. Beginning October 1, 1985, customary and prevailing charges will be updated each October 1.

(3) Beginning July 1, 1984, fee schedules will limit the reimbursement for diagnostic laboratory tests performed in independent laboratories, physicians' offices, and hospital laboratories for nonhospital patients. Initially the fees would be set on a statewide, regional, or carrierwide base. After three years, the payment will be based on a national fee schedule. At that time, lab services to hospital outpatients would revert back to being reimbursed on a reasonable cost basis.

FIGURE 3
SMI Monthly Per Capita Income

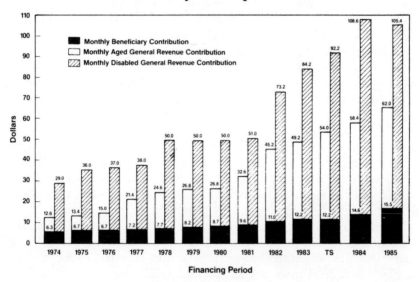

Financing Period: For periods 1983 and earlier, the financing period is July 1 through June 30. Transitional semester (TS), the financing period is July 1, 1983, through December 31, 1983. For 1984 and 1985 the financing period is January 1 through December 31.

Operations of the SMI Program—In calendar year 1984, 29.4 million people were covered under SMI. General revenue contributions during 1984 amounted to $17.1 billion, accounting for 73.6 percent of all SMI income. About 22.3 percent of all income resulted from the premiums paid by the participants, with interest payments to the SMI fund accounting for the remaining 4.1 percent. Of the $20.6 billion in SMI disbursements, $19.7 billion was for benefit payments while the remaining $0.9 billion was spent for administrative expenses. SMI administrative expenses were 4.3 percent of total disbursements. The historical operations of the SMI trust fund since calendar year 1978, as well as the projected operations of the fund for calendar years through 1987 for both alternative II-A and alternative II-B are shown in table 6. As can be seen, income has exceeded disbursements for most of the historical years, and the trust fund balance is projected to continue to increase through calendar year 1985 and then to decrease through calendar year 1987. As the report notes, the financial status of the program depends on both the total net assets and liabilities. It is, therefore, necessary to examine the incurred experience of the program, since it is this experience which is used to determine the actuarial rates discussed above and which forms the basis of the concept of actuarial soundness as it relates to the SMI program.

Actuarial Soundness of the SMI Program—The concept of actuarial soundness, as it applies to the supplementary medical insurance program, is closely related to the concept as it applies to private group insurance. The supplementary medical insurance program is essentially yearly renewable term insurance financed from premium income paid by the enrollees and from income contributed from general revenue in proportion to premium payments.

In testing the actuarial soundness of the supplementary medical insurance program, it is not appropriate to look beyond the period for which the enrollee premium rate and level of general revenue financing have been established. The primary tests of actuarial soundness, then, are that (1) income for years for which financing has been established be sufficient to meet the projected benefits and associated administrative expenses incurred for that period and (2) assets be sufficient to cover projected liabilities which will have been incurred by the end of the time but will not have been paid yet. Even if these tests of actuarial soundness are not met, the program can continue to operate if the trust fund remains at a level adequate to permit the payment of claims as presented. However, to protect against the possibility that cost increases under the program will be higher than assumed, assets should be sufficient to cover the impact of a moderate degree of projection error.

TABLE 6
SMI Fund Operations, Calendar Years 1978–1987
(In Billions)

Calendar Year	Total Income	Total Disbursements	Net Increase in Fund	Fund at End of Year
1978	$ 9.1	$ 7.8	$ 1.3	$ 4.4
1979	9.8	9.3	0.5	4.9
1980	10.9	11.2	−0.4	4.5
1981	15.4	14.0	1.3	5.9
1982	16.6	16.2	0.4	6.2
1983	19.8	19.0	0.8	7.1
1984	23.2	20.6	2.6	9.7
Alternative II-A:				
1985	24.9	23.5	1.3	11.0
1986	25.6	27.1	−1.5	9.5
1987	28.3	30.1	−1.9	7.6
Alternative II-B:				
1985	24.9	23.5	1.3	11.0
1986	25.6	27.1	−1.6	9.5
1987	28.3	30.2	−1.9	7.6

Note: Components may not add to totals due to rounding.

The primary tests for actuarial soundness and trust fund adequacy can be viewed by direct examination of absolute dollar levels. In providing an appropriate contingency or margin for error, however, there must be some relative measure. The relative measure or ratio used for this purpose is the ratio of net surplus or deficit to the following year's incurred expenditures. Figure 4 shows this ratio for historical years and for projected years under the intermediate assumptions (alternative II-B), as well as high and low cost sensitivity scenarios.

Financing for calendar year 1985 was established to reduce the excess of assets over liabilities to a more appropriate level. However, as experience has developed, it appears that this excess will be greater than expected at the time the calendar year 1985 financing was determined. As a result, the excess of assets over liabilities increases in the aggregate but only slightly when viewed as the ratio of the following 12-month projected incurred expenditures from December 31, 1984 to December 31, 1985.

132

FIGURE 4
Actuarial Status of the SMI Trust Fund

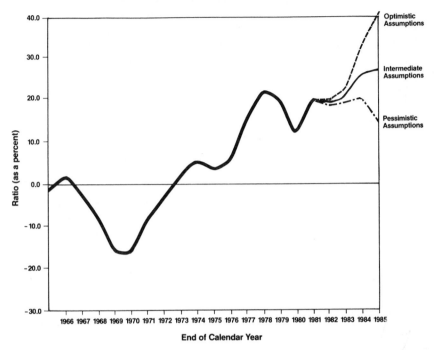

Note: The actuarial status of the SMI trust fund is measured by the ratio of the end-of-year surplus of deficit to the following year incurred expenditures.

Conclusion—The financing established through December 1985 is more than sufficient to cover projected benefit and administrative costs incurred through that time period, and to build a level of trust fund assets which is more than adequate to cover the impact of a moderate degree of projection error. The SMI program can thus be said to be actuarially sound; future financing needs to be established to reduce the excess to more appropriate levels.

Although the supplementary medical insurance program is financially sound, the board notes with concern the rapid growth in the cost of the program. The Board recommends that Congress take action to curtail the rapid growth in the supplementary medical insurance program.

133

Appendix D
Reducing the Deficit: Spending and Revenue Options, Congressional Budget Office 1985 Annual Report

(Following is a portion of the "Entitlements and Other Mandatory Spending" section from the report.)

This category presents 22 options that would either reduce outlays for entitlements and other mandatory spending or increase revenues earmarked to pay for these programs. ENT-1 through ENT-12 [presented here] deal with health care programs. ENT-13 through ENT-16 discuss alternatives for reducing net federal outlays for Social Security and other retirement and disability programs. ENT-17 through ENT-22 deal with other entitlements, including non-means-tested and partially means-tested benefits, means-tested benefits, and grants to state and local governments.

Several of the options are substitutes for one another. Also, in some instances, the individual summaries describe more than one specific policy alternative. The savings from the separate options—or from the variants within a single option—cannot be added together to arrive at a total.

All estimates of outlay savings and revenue gains from these options are calculated relative to the CBO baseline budget projection. The baseline projections assume CBO's short-run economic forecast and longer-run projections, as described in its report, *The Economic and Budget Outlook: Fiscal Years 1986–1990*. Baseline spending projections for entitlements and other mandatory spending programs reflect forecast changes in caseloads and in the average federal cost per beneficiary resulting, for example, from cost-of-living adjustments in benefit payments or increases in either the price of medical services or the intensity of their use.

Employees do not pay taxes on income received as employer-paid health care coverage [ENT-01]. This exclusion will reduce 1986 income tax revenues by approximately $17.0 billion. This form of income also escapes payroll taxation, costing the Social Security trust funds an additional $6.6 billion in lost 1986 revenues.

One option for limiting the exclusion would be to treat as taxable income in 1986 any portion of employer contributions exceeding $175 a month for family coverage and $70 a month for individuals, with

Tax Some Employer-Paid Health Insurance

Addition to CBO Baseline	Annual Added Revenues (Billions of Dollars)					Cumulative Five-Year Addition
	1986	1987	1988	1989	1990	
Income Tax	3.5	5.7	6.9	8.6	10.5	35.3
Payroll Tax	1.4	2.2	2.8	3.5	4.2	14.1

the amount indexed to reflect price increases. About 21 percent of income tax filing units would have been affected by a similar limit in 1984. The Congress has already adopted a similar approach with employer-paid group life insurance. The proposal would raise income tax revenues by $3.5 billion and payroll tax revenues by $1.4 billion in 1986. Over the 1986–1990 period, the revenue increases would amount to $35.3 billion and $14.1 billion, respectively. "Grandfathering" of current high-cost health insurance plans would reduce these amounts.

Both health-policy and tax-policy arguments have been made for limiting this exclusion. The exclusion leads to what many consider to be overly extensive health insurance coverage, which has expanded use of health care services unnecessarily and, consequently, driven up their prices. Moreover, the provision disproportionately benefits people with higher incomes, both because they tend to have somewhat larger employer-paid health insurance premiums that are excluded from taxation and because they are in higher marginal tax brackets. The average annual tax benefit from excluding employer-paid health insurance premiums in 1984 for tax filers with incomes between $10,000 and $15,000 is estimated at $85; for tax filers with incomes between $50,000 and $100,000, it is $641.

Opponents argue that even those people with the most extensive coverage are not covered excessively and that changing the current policy would lower their insurance coverage; this might, in turn, cause some of them to forgo some forms of medical care. They further argue that a uniform ceiling would have uneven effects, since a given employer's contribution purchases different levels of coverage depending on such factors as geographic location and the demographic characteristics of the firm's work force.

The Social Security Amendments of 1983 established a prospective payment system (PPS) that provides hospitals with strong incentives to reduce costs [ENT-02]. Under the new system, payment rates are set in advance for each of 468 diagnostic categories, known as diag-

Reduce Hospital Reimbursements Under Medicare

Savings from CBO Baseline	Annual Savings (Millions of Dollars)					Cumulative Five-Year Savings
	1986	1987	1988	1989	1990	
Limit Increases in Medicare's Prospective Payment Rates						
Budget Authority	−90	−280	−510	−810	−1,180	−2,870
Outlays	1,500	2,150	2,500	2,850	3,300	12,300
Reduce Medicare's Payments for Indirect Medical Education Costs						
Budget Authority	−20	−55	−110	−170	−260	−615
Outlays	310	430	580	650	720	2,700
Reduce Medicare's Payments for Direct Medical Education Expenses						
Budget Authority	−15	−40	−70	−100	−150	−375
Outlays	240	270	300	330	370	1,500

Note: Budget authority for the Hospital Insurance component of the Medicare program reflects all sources of income to the trust fund, including interest earned on reserves. Therefore, options that would reduce outlays also would allow reserves and interest income to increase. This accounts for the different arithmetic sign of budget authority and outlays in some of the entries.

nosis related groups (DRGs). Hospitals bear the burden if their costs exceed the fixed DRG payments, and they retain the surplus if their costs are lower. During the three-year phase-in period (fiscal years 1984–1986), prices will be based in part on prospective hospital-specific rates, in part on 18 regional rates (separate urban and rural rates for each of nine census regions), and in part on a single national urban or national rural rate. The final system will have only national urban and rural rates. Under the PPS, additional payments are made to hospitals for patients whose length of hospital stay or costs are unusually high, and for indirect medical education costs. The PPS rates currently do not cover capital-related costs (depreciation, interest, and rent) and direct medical education costs (residents' stipends, teachers' salaries, and administrative costs), which are reimbursed under a "reasonable cost" system.

Hospital reimbursements under Medicare might be reduced in the future in several ways: limit increases in Medicare's prospective payment rates; reduce Medicare's payments for indirect medical education costs; and reduce Medicare's payments for direct medical education costs.

Limit Increases in Medicare's Prospective Payment Rates—Beginning in 1987, Medicare's prospective payment rates to hospitals will be adjusted annually at the discretion of the Secretary of Health and Human Services. The 1986 adjustment will also be made by the Secretary but by law cannot exceed the growth rate in prices of goods and services purchased by hospitals (known as the market basket) plus one-quarter of a percentage point. The CBO baseline assumes the Secretary will allow annual increases equal to this limit in 1986 and in following years.

If the Congress froze the 1986 payment rates at their 1985 levels and limited future increases in the Medicare payment rate to the changes in the hospital market basket—not allowing the extra one-quarter of a percentage point—the savings through 1990 would be $12.3 billion. Moreover, restricting the increase would give hospitals greater incentives to become more efficient and to avoid procedures that are unnecessary or of limited value.

On the other hand, although admissions actually dropped in 1984, in the long run hospitals would have incentives to make up for the reduced Medicare revenue by admitting more patients, raising outpatient fees, and charging more to non-Medicare patients. Hospitals with predominantly Medicare patient populations might be forced to cut back services or close. Finally, high-cost beneficial advances in medical treatment might not be available to Medicare patients.

Reduce Medicare's Payments for Indirect Medical Education Costs—The prospective payment system includes higher payment rates to cover the additional patient care costs (that is, costs of treating each Medicare case) incurred by hospitals with teaching programs. These costs are known as indirect medical education costs. Hospitals with approved medical education programs receive an addition of 11.59 percent to the DRG portion of their payment for each 0.1 increase in the hospital's ratio of full-time equivalent interns and residents to its number of beds. This addition is double the estimate by the Health Care Financing Administration (HCFA) that a 0.1 increase in that ratio increases the cost of a Medicare case by approximately 5.8 percent. If this adjustment were reduced to 8.7 percent beginning in fiscal year 1986—halfway between the current statutory adjustment and the HCFA estimate—five-year savings would approach $2.7 billion.

The major argument for reducing the indirect medical education payments is that the current double adjustment factor overcompensates for any effect that a teaching program has on a hospital's costs for patient care. Hospitals may respond to this adjustment by substituting interns and residents for other medical personnel in a way that might not otherwise occur given relative wages and levels of productivity in providing patient care.

The issue of indirect medical education costs is very complex, however, and a uniform reduction may at best be a short-term solution. Many contend that the indirect teaching adjustment serves as a proxy to compensate for a number of factors that may legitimately increase costs—severity of illness of patients and inner-city locations of large teaching hospitals, for example—that are not adequately accounted for by the current DRG prices. Moreover, it is difficult to distinguish from these factors the effects that teaching programs have on costs of patient care. Finally, others argue that teaching hospitals provide the bulk of uncompensated and charity care to indigent patients, and that limiting the indirect teaching payments could reduce their ability to provide this care.

Reduce Medicare's Payment for Direct Medical Education Expenses— The direct costs of graduate medical education, which are currently excluded from the PPS, are reimbursed in proportion to the share of each hospital's total cost generated by Medicare patients. If this passthrough of direct medical education costs to Medicare were reduced by 25 percent beginning in fiscal year 1986, five-year savings would be approximately $1.5 billion.

There are several arguments for limiting this passthrough, which currently pays for nearly one-third of the direct costs of graduate medical education. First, other federal programs that subsidize medical education have been cut back in recent years because of an expected surplus of physicians and budgetary constraints. Second, the current system encourages expanding the direct costs of residency programs; reducing the level of reimbursement would lower—and might reverse—this incentive. Finally, some argue that the Hospital Insurance payroll tax is an inappropriate source of medical education subsidies, since those who benefit will generally earn incomes far higher than employees who pay the tax.

There are several drawbacks to reducing the direct medical education passthrough, however. First, because medical residents provide care to Medicare beneficiaries, setting a fair limit on the passthrough might be difficult. Few data are available to estimate the proportion of medical education costs that cover patient care. If the passthrough rate were set too low, other payers might be forced to subsidize care for Medicare patients since the current DRG prices do not reflect the costs of patient care provided by residents. Second, fewer physicians may be trained if hospitals responded to lower Medicare payments by cutting the size of the residency programs. While this might be desirable in those specialties experiencing the largest surplus, it could restrict training of physicians in other areas such as primary care. Finally, hospitals might decide to cut costs by reducing residents' salaries, thereby lowering their incomes during this portion of their training.

Medicare currently reimburses physicians under the Supplementary Medical Insurance (SMI) program for "reasonable" charges for all covered services [ENT-03]. A reasonable charge for a given service is the lowest of the physician's actual charge, the physician's customary charge for that service, and the prevailing charge for that service in the local community. This is known as the customary, prevailing, and reasonable (CPR) system.

Since the mid-1970s, the allowed rate of increase in prevailing fees has been limited to the rate of increase in an economywide index of office expenses and earnings—the Medicare economic index (MEI). The rate of increase in allowed fees has exceeded the MEI, though, because not all physicians' customary fees are at the ceiling set by prevailing fees. (About 60 percent of claim dollars were at the ceiling in July 1984.) Under the Deficit Reduction Act, physicians' allowed fees under Medicare were frozen for 15 months through September 30, 1985. This was accomplished by eliminating the update of both prevailing and customary fees that would otherwise have occurred on July 1, 1984, and by delaying until October 1, 1985, the update that would have occurred in July 1985.

The current freeze could be extended for another year, until October 1, 1986. Savings would be $490 million in 1986, and $3.2 billion through 1990. (These estimates assume a return to the CPR system in fiscal year 1987 and an update of all customary fees at that time. Prevailing fees, however, which were last adjusted in July 1983, would

ENT-03
Extend Freeze on Physicians' Fees Paid by Medicare for One More Year

Savings from CBO Baseline	Annual Savings (Millions of Dollars)					Cumulative Five-Year Savings
	1986	1987	1988	1989	1990	
Budget Authority	540	620	710	770	770	3,410
Outlays	490	560	650	740	740	3,180

increase only by the increase in the MEI during fiscal year 1986. Estimates for 1987 and beyond would, of course, be different if more far-reaching changes in physicians' reimbursement were enacted at that time.)

This option would generate savings relative to current law, while giving the Congress additional time to develop an alternative to the CPR system. Out-of-pocket costs for Medicare beneficiaries would not increase during the period of the freeze at least, since the current law effectively freezes physicians' charges to Medicare patients as well as Medicare's reimbursement rates. (Litigation now under way will determine whether extension of this freeze on physicians' charges is possible.) On the other hand, extending the freeze would mean that allowed fees under Medicare will have been unchanged since July 1983 for all physicians, even those with relatively low fees, while their costs have risen. This could increase reluctance of physicians to treat Medicare patients.

One alternative would be to modify the freeze by updating customary fees only for those physicians who were "participating physicians"—that is, who agreed to accept assignment for all their Medicare patients—during fiscal year 1985. (By accepting assignment, physicians agree to accept Medicare's allowed rates; patients are not billed for any excess of submitted charges over the allowed rates.) There would be no update on prevailing fees or on customary fees for nonparticipating physicians. Under this option, savings would be $390 million for 1986 and $2.9 billion over the five-year period. This would reward participating physicians by allowing their Medicare payment rates to increase if their customary fees are lower than prevailing fees in their community. Further, it would reduce the current variation in the rate that Medicare pays for a given service, making it less disruptive to implement uniform payment rates later as part of any major changes in the system.

ENT-04
Adopt a Fee Schedule for Reimbursing Physicians Under Medicare

Savings from CBO Baseline	Annual Savings (Millions of Dollars)					Cumulative Five-Year Savings
	1986	1987	1988	1989	1990	
Budget Authority	540	780	1,000	1,300	1,600	5,220
Outlays	490	650	890	1,200	1,400	4,630

As discussed in ENT-03, fees for physicians under Medicare's Supplementary Medical Insurance program have been frozen through September 30, 1985. As an alternative to continuing the current freeze or returning to the customary, prevailing, and reasonable (CPR) method of fee determination, a fee schedule based on the nationwide average of allowed amounts for each procedure—with adjustment for local differences in costs—could be put in place in October 1985 [ENT-04]. The fee schedule that would be effective from October 1, 1985, through September 30, 1986, could be set by average amounts allowed for each procedure during the previous year, with annual increases thereafter determined by the rate of increase in the Medicare economic index (MEI). Savings under this option—if fully implemented in October 1985—would be $490 million for 1986, and would total $4.6 billion over the five-year period, 1986–1990. Alternatively, this change could be phased in, for example, by freezing fees that are now higher than they would be under the new schedule until the new schedule caught up. Physician acceptance of the fee schedule might be enhanced, but savings would be lower.

Under the first approach, physicians with low fees would receive higher payment rates in fiscal year 1986, while physicians with high fees would have lower payment rates than previously. Savings for 1986 would be the same as if the current freeze were continued, but savings would be larger in later years because fee increases initiated by physicians would no longer directly affect Medicare reimbursements. Fees paid by Medicare would increase only in response to increases in physicians' office expenses or to higher national earnings per capita.

One problem with a fee schedule, however, is that a schedule based on average allowed amounts would incorporate elements of the current fee structure that many believe need to be corrected, such as more generous payments for inpatient services relative to similar care provided in physicians' offices, and excessive payments for certain procedures that are either ineffective or far less costly to perform now than when they were first introduced. Another problem is that control of costs probably requires constraints on volume of services provided as well as on fees. Although modification to the rate structure and the introduction of volume controls could be made incrementally following implementation, an alternative would be to delay major reform of physician payment methods until further studies are completed.

Medicare's Supplementary Medical Insurance program is partially funded by monthly premiums—currently $15.50—paid by benefici-

Increase Medicare's Premium for Physicians' Services

Savings from CBO Baseline	Annual Savings (Millions of Dollars)					Cumulative Five-Year Savings
	1986	1987	1988	1989	1990	
Budget Authority	1,650	2,550	3,300	4,300	5,400	17,200
Outlays	1,650	2,550	3,300	4,300	5,400	17,200

aries [ENT-05]. Between 1972 and 1982, premium receipts covered a declining share of SMI costs—dropping from 50 percent to 25 percent—because premiums were tied to the rate of growth in Social Security benefits, which is based on the Consumer Price Index, rather than to the faster-rising per capita cost of SMI. In 1982, premiums were set through 1985 (later extended through 1987) to cover 25 percent of the average benefits for an elderly enrollee. Under current law, beginning in 1988 the premium calculation will again be limited to the rate of growth of Social Security benefits. If, instead, the premium were set so that participants would pay 35 percent of benefits beginning January 1, 1986, and for all years thereafter, savings would total $1.7 billion in fiscal year 1986 and $17.2 billion over the five-year period. The estimated premium would be $24.30 on January 1, 1986, instead of the scheduled $17.30. These estimates incorporate the provision in current law that limits the application of a scheduled premium increase when it would exceed the dollar value of a person's cost-of-living increase under Social Security.

Under this option, the increase in payments would be shared by all enrollees, in contrast to other alternatives that affect only the users of medical services, who may be more financially pressed during the period of illness. Also, it would not affect the poorest since they are likely to be eligible for Medicaid, which usually pays the SMI premium on their behalf. For those not eligible for Medicaid, the higher premium would be about 5 percent of the average monthly Social Security benefit in 1986, slightly more of a burden than in 1967—the first full year for Medicare—when the premium was 3.6 percent of the average Social Security benefit.

Some current enrollees would find the increased premium burdensome, however. Some might drop SMI coverage and either do without care or turn to sources of free or reduced-cost care, which would increase demands on local governments. One alternative would be to raise gradually the share of benefits financed by premiums, increasing it from 25 percent to 35 percent over a five-year period. This phased

143

increase would lessen the burden on beneficiaries, but would reduce five-year federal savings to $12 billion. Another alternative would be a supplementary income-related premium, discussed in ENT-06.

Part B of Medicare offers Supplementary Medical Insurance (SMI), which covers a portion of enrollees' physician and other nonhospital charges. Participation is voluntary, and enrollees currently pay a monthly premium of $15.50. The premium is adjusted annually to cover 25 percent of the average costs incurred by an elderly enrollee. The balance of costs, nearly $20 billion for 1986, is paid from general revenues.

An alternative to increasing the share of costs financed by the current premium—which might reduce enrollment among lower-income beneficiaries—would be to impose a supplementary income-related premium. This could be most conveniently introduced through the income tax system, to avoid having to set up a new bureaucracy to collect means-tested premiums from enrollees.

A 1 percent tax could be imposed on enrollees' taxable income. A ceiling on added tax liability for each tax unit (usually the household) could be set by the number of SMI enrollees in the unit times the average value of subsidized SMI benefits per enrollee, so that no unit would pay more than the full actuarial value of its benefits. If an SMI tax of 1 percent were imposed on taxable income for all units with at least one SMI enrollee during the tax year, revenues earmarked for the SMI trust fund would be increased by $0.1 billion in 1986, and by $2.1 billion over the five-year period.

Although this approach would increase tax liabilities for a substantial proportion of SMI enrollees, the poorest enrollees—those with no taxable income—would not be affected. For those with taxable income, the percent increase in their tax liability—but not the dollar amount of the tax increase—would be larger for lower income people. Some might consider the tax inequitable since the amount of tax paid by each tax unit would not vary with the number of SMI

ENT-06
Use the Tax System to Impose a Supplementary Income-Related Premium for Physicians' Services

	Annual Added Revenues (Billions of Dollars)					Cumulative Five-Year Addition
	1986	1987	1988	1989	1990	
Addition to CBO Baseline	0.1	0.4	0.5	0.5	0.6	2.1

enrollees in a unit except for a small number of high-income tax units affected by the ceiling.

Eligibility for Hospital Insurance (HI) benefits is based on working-year tax contributions, half of which are paid by employees from after-tax income and half by employers from pre-tax income [ENT-07]. Eligibility for Supplementary Medical Insurance (SMI) depends on payment of a premium, which currently covers about 25 percent of SMI benefits. Hence, 50 percent of the insurance value of HI benefits and 75 percent of the insurance value of SMI benefits might be treated as taxable income for enrollees, effective January 1, 1986, with the resulting tax proceeds returned to the Medicare trust funds. This proposal is analogous to the taxation of Social Security benefits, which is already part of the law for beneficiaries with incomes exceeding $25,000 (for individuals) or $32,000 (for couples).

If the current income thresholds for the tax on Social Security benefits were used to limit the application of the tax on Medicare benefits, too—with taxable Medicare benefits added to taxable Social Security benefits to compare to the threshold—taxing both HI and SMI benefits would yield additional revenues of $0.5 billion in 1986 and $9.3 billion over the five-year period 1986–1990. If no income thresholds were used to limit the application of the Medicare tax, additional revenues would be $0.7 billion in 1986 and $11.2 billion over the five-year period.

A tax on HI benefits would strengthen the HI trust fund. A tax on SMI benefits would shift some SMI costs from the general taxpayer to beneficiaries without increasing costs for low-income beneficiaries and thereby not threatening their access to care. Benefits provided to Medicare enrollees would not be reduced. Since this option would use the mechanism already in place for taxing Social Security benefits, it would present no additional administrative difficulty.

On the other hand, because of their better health, people with higher incomes are typically less costly to the Medicare program, so that requiring them to pay a relatively greater share of the costs might

ENT-07
Tax a Portion of Medicare Benefits

	Annual Added Revenues (Billions of Dollars)					Cumulative Five-Year Addition
	1986	1987	1988	1989	1990	
Addition to CBO Baseline	0.5	1.8	2.1	2.3	2.6	9.3

be viewed as inequitable by some. If the income thresholds were eliminated, tax liabilities for elderly couples with taxable income would increase by $350 to $1,500 in 1986. Further, unlike the tax on Social Security benefits, this tax would be imposed on the insurance value of in-kind benefits rather than on dollar benefits actually received—a modification of current tax policy. Finally, some might object to this tax because enrollees could not alter their tax liability by choosing a different package of benefits, except by dropping SMI coverage altogether.

Appreciable federal savings in Medicare's Supplementary Medical Insurance program could be realized by increasing the deductible—that is, the amount that beneficiaries must pay for services each year before the government shares responsibility [ENT-08]. The deductible is now $75 a year. This deductible has been increased only twice since Medicare began in 1966, when it was set at $50. Hence, the deductible has fallen relative to average per capita benefits from 70 percent in 1967 to an estimated 10 percent for 1985. Increasing the SMI deductible to $200 on January 1, 1986, and indexing it thereafter to the rate of growth in the Consumer Price Index would save $610 million in fiscal year 1986 and $6 billion over the five-year period 1986–1990.

Such an increase would spread the burden of reduced federal outlays across most beneficiaries, raising their out-of-pocket costs by no more than $125 each in 1986. Since a larger proportion of beneficiaries would not exceed the deductible (currently about 35 percent do not), there would be more beneficiaries with maximal incentives for prudent consumption of medical care, and administrative costs to process claims also could be reduced.

On the other hand, even relatively small increases in out-of-pocket costs could prove burdensome to low-income beneficiaries who do not qualify for Medicaid. That might, in turn, discourage some people from seeking needed care.

Under current law, physicians' services and hospital outpatient care are reimbursed under the Supplementary Medical Insurance

ENT-08
Increase Medicare's Deductible for Physician Services

Savings from CBO Baseline	Annual Savings (Millions of Dollars)					Cumulative Five-Year Savings
	1986	1987	1988	1989	1990	
Budget Authority	850	1,200	1,400	1,500	1,750	6,700
Outlays	610	1,050	1,250	1,450	1,600	5,960

146

ENT-09
Increase Cost Sharing for Medicare
and Add Catastrophic Protection

Savings from CBO Baseline	Annual Savings (Millions of Dollars)					Cumulative Five-Year Savings
	1986	1987	1988	1989	1990	
Budget Authority	690	840	810	610	500	3,450
Outlays	1,710	2,760	3,230	3,740	4,250	15,690

(SMI) component of Medicare, while hospital, skilled nursing, and home health care services are reimbursed under the Hospital Insurance (HI) program [ENT-09]. Each program has its own financing, deductible, and cost-sharing provisions.

The HI and SMI components of Medicare could be better coordinated, with coverage expanded to provide a cap on out-of-pocket expenses for covered services under either part of Medicare. This catastrophic benefit could be entirely financed by a premium set for a new Part C of Medicare, which could be a required addition for those electing SMI coverage. A deductible of $200 could apply for all SMI services, with the amount indexed to the rate of growth in the Consumer Price Index (CPI). In addition, a deductible equal to the average cost of a hospital day (currently $400) could be required for each hospital admission, while eliminating all coinsurance payments for hospital stays. After the deductibles were met, coinsurance of 20 percent of costs could be required on all services except hospital stays, with beneficiaries' maximum annual liability for cost sharing through the HI and SMI deductible and coinsurance provisions limited to $2,000. This limit, too, could be indexed to the rate of growth in the CPI. If implemented on January 1, 1986, estimated savings under these combined provisions would total $1.7 billion in 1986, and $15.7 billion over the five-year period 1986–1990.

The prospective payment system for hospital reimbursement, while providing incentives to hospitals to limit extended stays by releasing patients as soon as they are well enough, may at the same time encourage multiple admissions or admissions for procedures or tests that could be done on an outpatient basis. Applying a per-admission deductible would reduce that potential problem by requiring patients to pay the full first-day costs for each admission. (Contrary to expectations, however, Medicare admissions did not increase in 1984.)

Requiring a coinsurance rate of 20 percent of daily costs for all services except hospital stays would simplify Medicare's cost-sharing provisions and would give enrollees an incentive lacking now to reduce their use of skilled nursing facilities and home health services. Total health care costs could decline because of reduced use of services induced by the higher copayments required of beneficiaries, although this decrease might be small since 75 percent to 80 percent of beneficiaries have supplemental coverage for copayments. Further, any decline in costs could be offset by potentially greater costs for patients who exceed the catastrophic cap. One longer-term benefit of a catastrophic cap might be to reduce the proportion of enrollees who purchase supplementary coverage, thereby eliminating their Medigap premium costs and increasing the effect of Medicare's cost-sharing provisions on reducing their demand for services.

Preliminary estimates indicate that total copayments would be virtually unchanged in 1986 under this option, equal to about $400 per enrollee. Copayments would increase for most enrollees not using hospital services during the year, however, and fewer than 1 percent of these enrollees would benefit from the cap on copayments. For enrollees admitted to the hospital, average copayments would fall. About 23 percent of enrollees using hospital services, and 5 percent of all enrollees, would benefit from the catastrophic cap in 1986. Although each enrollee's annual out-of-pocket costs for covered services would be capped at $2,000, enrollees would still be liable for disallowed charges, noncovered services, and premium costs.

The annual Medicare premium for 1986 would be about $200 for Part B, and about $75—or $6.25 monthly—for the new Part C. The Part C premium would be higher if benefits were expanded to include the costs of long hospital stays (over 150 days a year) and nursing facility stays (over 100 days), which are not currently covered by Medicare. The premium would also be higher if more services were used by enrollees who approached or exceeded the cap.

ENT-10
Tax Premiums for "Medigap" Policies

Addition to CBO Baseline	Annual Added Revenues (Millions of Dollars)					Cumulative Five-Year Addition
	1986	1987	1988	1989	1990	
Impose a 30-Percent Tax on Premiums for Medigap Policies	3,150	4,550	4,950	5,400	5,850	23,950

Over 60 percent of all Medicare participants purchase (or receive from employers) private coverage to supplement Medicare [ENT-10]. These plans—known as "Medigap" policies—reduce patients' out-of-pocket payments for Medicare's deductible amounts and coinsurance. Although the plans vary widely, they often pay all of the cost-sharing portions of Medicare (for example, the 20 percent coinsurance for physicians' charges). Consequently, people with Medigap coverage use services at a higher rate than those covered only by Medicare, yet Medicare pays most of the costs of these additional services (for example, 80 percent of physicians' reasonable charges).

To recoup the extra federal outlays arising from greater use of health care by holders of supplemental coverage, a tax of 30 percent could be imposed on premiums for Medigap policies that pay any part of the first $1,000 of Medicare's required cost sharing. This proposal would not affect the prevalence of insurance protection for unusually large health costs. Federal savings would stem both from the premium tax receipts and from a reduction in use of health care by those who would drop Medigap coverage or change the type of policy to avoid an increase in premiums. The additional revenues, which could be dedicated to the two Medicare trust funds, plus the outlay reductions would total $3.2 billion in 1986 and $24 billion over the 1986–1990 period.

This option would lead to more equal federal aid for all participants by requiring those with Medigap coverage to bear the additional costs they impose on Medicare. Moreover, the reduced use of services might help to slow the growth in health care costs. Finally, very low-income elderly and disabled people would not be affected, since Medicaid pays their deductible amounts and coinsurance.

The premium tax would, however, increase the cost of the current type of Medigap policies and therefore discourage their purchase. Some who would otherwise have purchased supplemental coverage would have trouble meeting out-of-pocket costs during a year of unusually high medical expenditures. Without Medigap coverage, beneficiaries could pay as much as $1,000 in cost sharing, which could represent a substantial portion of their incomes.

The Hospital Insurance (HI) component of Medicare, which accounts for almost 70 percent of total program outlays, is financed by a portion of the Social Security payroll tax [ENT-11]. Employees covered by the HI program and their employers currently each contribute 1.35 percent of the first $39,600 of earnings. The tax rate is scheduled to increase to 1.45 percent in 1986, and the taxable earnings ceiling rises automatically with average wages.

ENT-11
Increase the Hospital Insurance Payroll Tax

Addition to CBO Baseline	Annual Added Revenues (Millions of Dollars)					Cumulative Five-Year Addition
	1986	1987	1988	1989	1990	
Increase Payroll Tax Rates by Half a Percentage Point	13,900	19,000	20,500	22,000	23,600	99,000

Increasing the HI payroll tax rate would reduce the federal budget deficit and help maintain the solvency of the HI trust fund, which is projected to be depleted in the mid-1990s. A 0.5 percentage-point increase in the tax rate for both employers and employees beginning in 1986 would generate $99 billion in revenues over the 1986–1990 period, and would delay depletion of the trust fund.

Some argue, however, that payroll taxes are already too high. Currently scheduled increases mean that the combined employer and employee Social Security tax rate—for retirement benefits, disability payments, and Medicare—will have increased by 3.6 percentage points between 1975 and 1990, from 11.7 percent to 15.3 percent. Moreover, Social Security payroll taxes already account for an increasing share of total federal revenues—rising from 26 percent in 1980 to about 34 percent in 1989. Further increases in the payroll tax could have adverse effects on employment and inflation, because the cost of hiring workers would rise. In addition, this option would increase both the relative and absolute tax burden of those with lower earnings, because the tax applies only to earnings below a specified limit.

Appreciable savings could be realized by transforming Medicaid's funding for long-term care services into a block grant [ENT-12]. States would have to match the federal grant based on current rates, and for

ENT-12
Limit Payments for Long-Term Care Services Through a Block Grant

Savings from CBO Baseline	Annual Savings (Millions of Dollars)					Cumulative Five-Year Savings
	1986	1987	1988	1989	1990	
Budget Authority	850	1,150	1,450	1,750	2,100	7,300
Outlays	850	1,150	1,450	1,750	2,100	7,300

the first year each state would receive the 1985 amount. After 1986, federal grants could reflect adjustments relative to state population and other factors, such as the probable use of service in an area, the number of poor elderly and disabled people in the state, and a per capita payment for each type of service adjusted for the local costs of long-term care services. Increases in total federal payments, however, would be limited to the inflation rate for medical care. Federal savings over the next five years could accrue to $7.3 billion.

Advocates of such a plan believe that it would encourage states to service their long-term care patients more cost-effectively. Given more flexibility in the use of funds, states would be encouraged to substitute lower-cost services, such as home and community-based care, for costly services, such as institutionalizing all mentally ill or mentally retarded patients for long periods.

Opponents of a block grant for long-term care fear that too much responsibility and financial burden would be shifted to the states. They believe that if federal funding is decreased, some needed services would not be provided because some states would not provide supplemental funding. To provide adequate and quality care, some states would have to either increase local taxes or perhaps reduce some benefits to the less-poor beneficiary population. Others suggest that some states might respond to the plan by increasing the use of acute-care services that would still be partially funded by the federal government.

An additional option would be to fold current funding for long-term care under the Social Services Block Grant (SSBG) into the new grant. While the exact amount of SSBG funds used this way by each state would have to be estimated, one program instead of two would likely be administratively superior. States would allocate resources from a single agency and would delegate to local agencies or contractors the necessary screening of and health care planning for patients.

Index